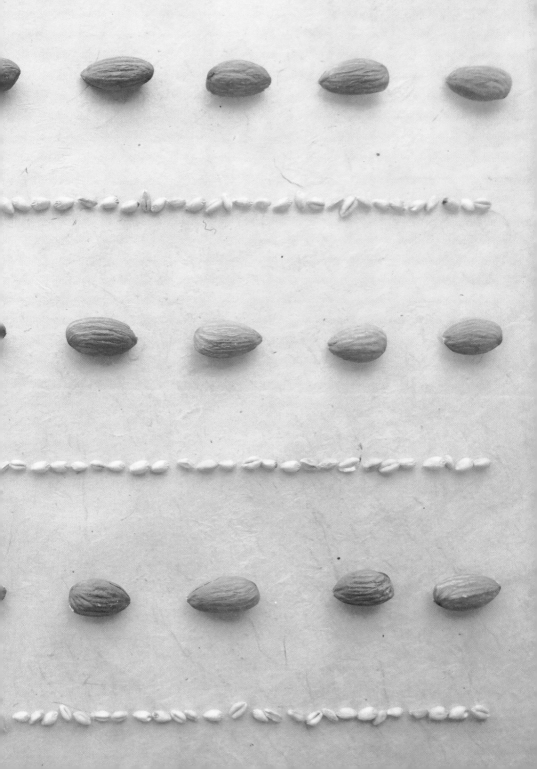
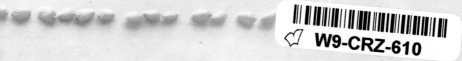

W9-CRZ-610

Gandhi's Search
for the Perfect Diet

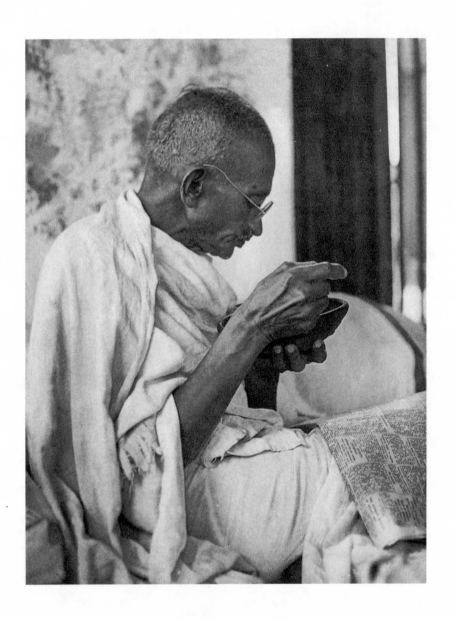

Gandhi's Search for the Perfect Diet

EATING WITH THE

WORLD IN MIND

Nico Slate

UNIVERSITY OF WASHINGTON PRESS

Seattle

A Capell Family Book

The Capell Family Endowed Book Fund supports the publication of books that deepen the understanding of social justice through historical, cultural, and environmental studies.

UNIVERSITY OF WASHINGTON PRESS
www.washington.edu/uwpress

LIBRARY OF CONGRESS CATALOGING-IN-PUBLICATION DATA
Names: Slate, Nico, author.
Title: Gandhi's search for the perfect diet : eating with the world in mind / Nico Slate.
Description: Seattle : University of Washington Press, [2019] | Series: Global South Asia | Includes bibliographical references and index. |
Identifiers: LCCN 2018026828 (print) | LCCN 2018047384 (ebook) | ISBN 9780295744971 (ebook) | ISBN 9780295744957 (hardcover : alk. paper)
Subjects: LCSH: Food preferences. | Food—Quality. | Diet—History. | Public health.
Classification: LCC TX353 (ebook) | LCC TX353 .S53 2019 (print) | DDC 613.2—dc23
LC record available at https://lccn.loc.gov/2018026828

FRONTISPIECE: Mahatma Gandhi, a.k.a. Mohandas Karamchand Gandhi (1869–1948), photographed in Gujarat, India, on April 6, 1930. Sueddeutsche Zeitung Photo / Alamy Stock Photo.

For the mango, the papaya, and the pomegranate

By their fruit you will recognize them. Do people pick grapes from thornbushes, or figs from thistles? Likewise, every good tree bears good fruit.

MATTHEW 7:15

Contents

Photo gallery follows page 118

Acknowledgments

My mother, Karena Slate, worked late. A single mother who commuted sixty miles to teach in a public school, she did not have much time to cook. Around the age of twelve, I began to prepare meals for my mom and for myself. No matter how simple the meal—a spaghetti sauce spiced only with salt and pepper, a "soup" that was nothing but water and boiled vegetables—my mom always raved about my culinary genius. My love for cooking owes everything to her kindness.

Therese Tardio, Matt Coffman, and Jonathan Nassim all spent hours discussing Gandhi's diet with me. My colleagues and students at Carnegie Mellon University challenged me to think more critically about Gandhi's struggles with food. Several anonymous readers offered sharp and insightful comments. John Soluri read the manuscript and suggested dozens of improvements. Lorri Hagman of the University of Washington Press was generous and supportive throughout the process, and offered thoughtful suggestions on nearly every page of the manuscript. Anne Mathews copyedited the manuscript with great care and skill, and Julie Van Pelt guided me (and the book) through the production process. Apoorv Bajaj, Haribhai Mori, Mahendra Phate, and all my friends at the Kamalnayan Jamnalal Bajaj Foundation offered hospitality and inspiration. My brother, Peter Slate, taught me to believe in myself. Emily Mohn-Slate read the manuscript, offered critical insights into its arguments, heroically put up with my cooking, and filled my days with poetry. Kai Slate and Lucia Slate helped me make pumpkin pudding, ate my gorilla munch, and sometimes even asked for more. My deepest thanks to all.

Timeline of Gandhi's Life with Food

1869   Born on October 2 into a vegetarian family in Porbandar, India

1883   Marries at the age of thirteen to Kasturba Makanji Kapadia

1885–87 Experiments with eating meat in order to compete with "the mighty Englishman"

1888   Sails for London after vowing to avoid "women, wine, and meat"

1890   Joins the London Vegetarian Society

1891   Publishes his first article in the *Vegetarian*; criticizes the taxation of salt

1893   Arrives in South Africa; experiments with a twelve-day raw food diet

1904   Establishes the Phoenix Settlement—first major effort to grow his own food

1905   Declares that the salt tax "should be immediately abolished"

1906   Mobilizes resistance to anti-Asian racism in South Africa

1908   Jailed for the first time; protests prison food and denounces mealie pap, in particular, as not "suitable for the Asiatic constitution"

1909   Embraces mealie pap as "a sweet and strength-giving food"

1910   Founds Tolstoy Farm

1911   Begins a "saltless" diet; writes a friend, "I see death in chocolates"

1912   Eliminates all dairy products from his diet

1913   Publishes a recipe for almond milk; fasts in response to his son's affair with a married woman

1914	Vows to never consume milk or ghee
1915	Returns to India and founds the Sabarmati Ashram
1918	Begins drinking goat's milk after contracting dysentery
1919	Fasts to protest the Jallianwala Bagh Massacre
1920	Launches the Noncooperation Movement with a day of fasting and prayer; writes a friend hoping to share "some luscious mangoes"
1924	Fasts for Hindu-Muslim unity
1929	Experiments with a monthlong raw food diet; receives a peanut milk recipe from George Washington Carver
1930	Launches the Salt March
1932	Fasts against the Communal Award
1934	Founds the All-India Village Industries Association
1936	Establishes the Sevagram Ashram
1941	Eats mangoes meant for others and declares, "Mango is a cursed fruit"
1942	Launches the Quit India movement
1946	Sends message to Vallabhbhai Patel, Rajendra Prasad, and Jagjivan Ram: "Abolish salt tax, remember Dandi March"
1947	Fasts for peace in Calcutta
1948	Fasts for peace in Delhi; assassinated on January 30

Gandhi's Search
for the Perfect Diet

INTRODUCTION

The Scale

For men like me, you have to measure them not by the rare
moments of greatness in their lives, but by the amount of dust they
collect on their feet in the course of life's journey.

MAHATMA GANDHI, 1947

IN 1931, FRENCH CUSTOMS OFFICIALS DETAINED MOHANDAS KARAM-
chand Gandhi in the coastal town of Marseilles. Asked to declare his
belongings, Gandhi replied, "I am a poor mendicant. My earthly possessions consist of six spinning wheels, prison dishes, a can of goat's milk,
six homespun loincloths and towels, and my reputation which cannot
be worth much." On his way to meet the King of England and to parley
with the powerbrokers of the British Empire, Gandhi knew that his reputation was worth a great deal—far more than his meager belongings. He
also knew that his reputation depended on his scant possessions. His
power grew in proportion to his humility, to the meagerness of his things
and the slim body that carried them.[1]

Gandhi weighed about one hundred pounds. He stood five feet, six
inches tall. His body, renowned for its spare strength, symbolized his
humility, his nonviolence, and his identification with the poor. In his thin
but strong frame, he embodied one of his greatest passions—his diet.
Throughout his adult life, he thought about food, talked about food, and
experimented with food. Understanding Gandhi's diet is to understand
the man and his life, and to connect two of history's perennial questions:
how to live and what to eat.[2]

Gandhi embraced many of today's most popular dietary principles, especially calorie restriction and a diet high in fruits, nuts, and vegetables. He lived Michael Pollan's advice to "eat food, not too much, mostly plants." He fasted, made his own yogurt, spent months eating only raw food, and avoided salt, sweets, meat, and processed food. Some of his favorite foods drew upon the rich culinary traditions of India. As a young man, he relished the intricate blend of spices—coriander, cumin, ginger, turmeric, cardamom—that went into even the most basic dishes, such as *khichdi*, the lentil and rice staple that would remain one of his comfort foods. As he aged, he reduced his diet to an elemental core befitting the austere simplicity of the man those French customs officials found in Marseilles, the man whose body had become a global icon and a source of power.[3]

Gandhi's body was a text that different audiences read according to their own perspective. Indians waited hours to catch a fleeting glimpse of the mahatma as his train rolled by. They sought *darśan*, the religious viewing of a sacred idol. To such spectators, Gandhi's body was semi-divine. To Winston Churchill, by contrast, it was "alarming and also nauseating" to see Gandhi "striding half-naked up the steps of the Vice-regal Palace." Gandhi recognized the power of his image. His diet, however, had nothing to do with appearances. Given the centrality of his body to his public image, it is striking that he was unconcerned with the relationship between what he ate and how he looked.[4]

By nourishing his body, Gandhi cultivated the energy he needed to lead protracted nonviolent struggles. In his words, "The vigour of mind is possible only in a healthy body." Physical health was only one advantage of his diet. Gandhi saw a more profound connection between his body, his purpose, and his achievements. He viewed his body as a microcosm of the larger world. "We but mirror the world," he explained. "All the tendencies present in the outer world are to be found in the world of our body."[5]

Gandhi developed an ecological diet that respected the many connections between his food and his physical, social, and political environments. He redefined nutrition as a holistic approach to building a more just world. As nutritionists Geoffrey Cannon and Claus Leitzmann have written, "It is only by combining biological, social and environmental approaches that nutrition science can fulfill its potential to preserve, maintain, develop and sustain life on earth." Gandhi modeled such an integrated approach to nutrition. He ate with the world in mind.[6]

An ecological diet was the foundation of what the philosopher Akeel Bilgrami has called "Gandhi's integrity." Bilgrami distinguishes two facets of this integrity: the fact that Gandhi "tried to make his actions live up to his ideals," and the degree to which "his thought itself was highly integrated." Bilgrami is right that Gandhi's "ideas about very specific political strategies in specific contexts flowed (and in his mind necessarily flowed) from ideas that were very remote from politics." By grappling with the ethical and political dimensions of what he ate, Gandhi brought his values into the most elemental realms of human life. He embodied his integrity.[7]

Gandhi's life story reveals the power of food as a catalyst of personal and political transformation. As a young man, he rarely thought about what he ate; often, he ate too much. He also did not think a lot about changing the world. In 1888, when he left India to attend law school in London, his goal was a lucrative career. In London, he began to reform his diet and to develop a commitment to serving others. These changes were connected. His experiments with food planted the seeds of a profound revolution in his self-conception and his social commitments.[8]

From London, he traveled to South Africa to represent the interests of wealthy businessmen. Like his clients, he traveled first class, wore expensive suits, and ate lavishly. Twenty years later, he left South Africa wearing Indian clothes, identifying with the poor, and eating a simple diet of fruits, nuts, and whole grains. Gandhi's dietary evolution was a product of the personal and political upheaval that marked his time in London and in South Africa. But his diet was more than a product of his politics; his passion for food helped drive his politics.[9]

The pillars of his diet—vegetarianism, limiting salt and sweets, rejecting processed food, eating raw food, fasting—were all deeply connected to his politics and, in particular, to his conception of nonviolence or what he called *ahimsa*, an ancient Sanskrit word for "nonharm." Gandhi's embrace of *ahimsa* began with his vegetarianism and expanded to include a personal, political, and dietary commitment to what historian Aishwary Kumar calls "radical equality" and historian Ajay Skaria deems "unconditional equality." As Skaria argues, Gandhi's commitment to equality extended not just to people but also included "the absolute equality of all beings." Equality was at the core of his nonviolence—and of what he ate. Beginning in London and in South Africa, and continuing throughout his life, Gandhi pursued equality through his diet.[10]

Gandhi's dietary *ahimsa* reflected the transnational circuits of his life. As he sailed from India to London to South Africa, the borders of his world and of his diet expanded together. He sampled foods and recipes from throughout the world, and developed an expansive and experimental culinary cosmopolitanism. Many of the ideas and practices that defined his diet came to shape all facets of his politics: not just nonviolence, but also tolerance, humility, and relentless experimentation. These values were all linked. His dietary experiments taught Gandhi to be humble, and his humility drove his tolerance. His culinary cosmopolitanism grew alongside and helped inspire other forms of inclusivity—especially in regards to race, class, gender, and caste.[11]

Food scholar Anita Mannur cautions against "an easy culinary cosmopolitanism" that "flattens out the unevenness of multiculturalism." We must avoid celebrating the ability of elites to appropriate the foods and cultures of others. While recognizing such dangers, philosopher Uma Narayan writes that "a willingness to eat the food of Others seems to indicate at least a growing democracy of the palate." When does a democracy of the palate inspire other forms of democracy? The answer suggested by the history of Gandhi's diet concerns to what extent the eating of unfamiliar food is connected to other forms of social, political, and economic solidarity. His dietary transgressions inspired Gandhi to challenge other limitations in his thinking and his life. As he became a more expansive eater, he also became a more thoughtful and compassionate human being and a more effective advocate for justice. His diet fueled his purpose and his power. Food helped turn a man into a mahatma.[12]

The word *mahatma* means "great soul." The renowned poet Rabindranath Tagore gave Gandhi the title "Mahatma," a fitting tribute to a man who understood his life as a spiritual quest. "All religions," Gandhi wrote, "have looked upon this body as a place where one may meet and recognize God." Such divine recognition required seeing the body as a vehicle for public service. "This body is of some service," he believed, "only if it is well used, that is, made the abode of God." In his autobiography, he connected religious devotion to public service. "If I found myself entirely absorbed in the service of the community," he wrote, "the reason behind it was my desire for self-realization. I had made the religion of service my own, as I felt that God could be realized only through service." For Gandhi, public service was the way to God, and diet was central to service. Inspired by a spiritual quest for *moksha*, liberation from the confines of one's own ego, the mahatma sought in food a way to transcend himself in the service of others. But as his life makes clear, too much attention to diet can become a self-obsessive trap.[13]

Gandhi sought the perfect diet. He worried about what to eat as well as how much to eat, and his dietary anxiety reveals the risks of excessive concern with food. His fixation on food inspired an equally troublesome obsession with nutrition. Influenced by the discovery of vitamins, he succumbed to a nutrient mystique that has only grown stronger with time. Bombarded with claims about the latest supernutrient—whether omega-3 fatty acids, resveratrol, or lycopene—many consumers buy (literally) into what food scholar Gyorgy Scrinis has labeled "nutritionism." Eating has been reduced to a medical act. A fierce critic of consumerism, Gandhi would have decried what Scrinis has called the "deep complicity between nutritionism and the commercial interests of food manufacturers." By funding biased research studies, food companies promote a reductionist approach to nutrition that privileges processed items over fresh whole foods. Gandhi would be aghast. He lived through the early industrialization of food, and defended unprocessed food with his pen and his plate. Yet his embrace of nutritionism anticipated the tactics of the industrial giants he abhorred.[14]

Gandhi's quest for the perfect diet contributed to the most controversial dimension of his relationship to food—how little he ate. "While planning a diet," he wrote, "all of us should cut down on the quantity we consume." Even for the mahatma, eating less was not easy. He had to learn moderation. "There was a time," he reminisced, when he "would drink tea in the morning, have breakfast two or three hours later, a regular meal at one p.m., then tea at about three o'clock and a full meal between 6 and 7 in the evening." As a consequence of this "excessive" eating, "a medicine bottle was always at his side." By reducing his calories, he improved his health and found he had "three times the energy" to do good work in the world. As with many facets of his diet, Gandhi pursued calorie restriction to the extreme. His weight would give many doctors cause for concern. His height and weight gave him a body mass index (BMI) of 16.1, well under the standard target range of 18.5–24.9. How much to respect such numbers is an ongoing question, but regardless of whether Gandhi's weight was unhealthy, his drive to eat less reveals the dangers of compulsive self-denial.[15]

Gandhi's obsession with self-denial blunted the inclusivity of his culinary cosmopolitanism and turned his experiments with food into a compulsive focus on the self—a focus that is one of the hallmarks of eating disorders. He recognized the dark side of his dietary obsessions. When it came to food, he wrote, "I feel like making innocent experiments. Maybe there is some attachment in that." The tragedy of Gandhi's diet is that he recognized the dangers of dietary obsession and yet was unable to escape them.[16]

Gandhi's struggles sidestep some of the dietary neuroses that plague the modern world. He was obsessed with food, but not with his weight or his body image. He rejected the equation of health with a muscular build. "A healthy body," he told a friend, did not need to be "a weight-lifting body." You can search the ninety volumes of his collected works in vain for any reference to weight as the measure of his diet. For him, the scale that mattered did not weigh his body, but rather all the good he accomplished with his body.[17]

Food enriched all of Gandhi's life, but the same quest for integrity that inspired him to become a mahatma drove him toward dietary perfectionism. He struggled to care about food without caring too much, to be disciplined without being obsessive. His struggles were especially difficult when he tried to balance his role as nutritional expert with his position as a husband and a father.

On a Saturday in June 1914, a few months before the world erupted in war, Gandhi wrote his son, Manilal, to reassure him of his love. Gandhi had eliminated table salt from his diet and encouraged his loved ones to do the same, but Manilal had rejected his father's advice. While his opinion on salt was strong, Gandhi did not want his eating choices to trump his most vital priorities. He told his son, "I don't love you any the less for your not adopting a saltless diet." The fact that such reassurance was necessary speaks to the dangers of his dietary attachments, even those he tried to hold lightly. "There is no special sin or virtue in eating or not eating salt," he told his son. It was, after all, not the diet that mattered, but the meaning behind the diet. In his words, it was "the underlying principle" that "raises moral issues." The "moral issues" raised by salt would continue to challenge Gandhi's relationship with his family, even while inspiring one of the greatest civil disobedience campaigns in history, a campaign that began with an illegal pinch of salt from the Arabian sea.[18]

CHAPTER 1

Salt

What is life worth without trials and tribulations which are the salt
of life?

GANDHI, 1930

O N APRIL 6, 1930, GANDHI GATHERED A HANDFUL OF SALTY SAND
from a crowded beach on the west coast of India. With that simple
act, he shook the foundations of the British Empire. A few months earlier, the Indian National Congress had endorsed the goal of *purna swaraj,*
or "complete independence." Gandhi's challenge was to make that goal a
reality. He had numbers on his side, as British rule required the tacit support of India's millions. If enough Indians withdrew their support, the
British Raj would crumble. India's population was split along multiple
lines—religion, class, caste, and language—and the British used divide
and rule tactics to maintain their power. Gandhi needed a strategy that
could unite all Indians in opposition to British oppression. He found his
strategy in salt.

Everyone needs salt to survive. "Next to air and water," Gandhi
declared, "salt is perhaps the greatest necessity of life." From macaws to
moose, many animals travel miles to find salt licks and other natural
sources of salt. For much of human history, salt was a precious commodity, traded across deserts and seas. The word *salary* comes from the
Roman practice of giving soldiers a regular payment to purchase salt.
Wars were fought to control sources of salt, as they are for oil today. Salt
is no longer so precious; while some people struggle to buy their daily

salt, many consume large amounts, unaware of the salt packed into everything from bread to breakfast cereal. In the gap between those who have too little and those who have too much, Gandhi saw an opportunity to challenge the British Empire.[1]

In colonial India, the British maintained a monopoly on the collection and production of salt. The salt monopoly affected all Indians, but it especially hurt the poor. Even a slight increase in the price of salt harmed the millions of Indians with barely enough income to purchase food and other basic necessities. Gandhi deemed the salt monopoly a "curse" and set about to end it. He turned to nonviolent civil disobedience, or what he called *satyagraha*. From the Sanskrit for "holding firm to the truth," *satyagraha* communicated the resistance to injustice that Gandhi understood as the heart of nonviolence. Others called it "passive resistance," but there was nothing passive about *satyagraha*.[2]

In the spring of 1930, the sixty-year-old mahatma walked 240 miles from his ashram near the banks of the Sabarmati River to the coastal town of Dandi. The twenty-four-day journey—referred to as the Salt March or the Dandi March—captured the attention of the world. Gandhi had announced his intention to break the law by gathering natural salt from that most abundant source—the ocean. One man's defiance could not alone threaten British rule. By gathering a fistful of salty sand, Gandhi did more than challenge the British to arrest him; he appealed to his fellow Indians to join a nonviolent battle for freedom. He was not disappointed. Throughout India, protesters began to produce and distribute salt in open defiance of the law. The Salt Satyagraha had begun.[3]

Even as he championed greater access to salt, Gandhi limited his own intake and argued that many people consumed too much. Fruits, vegetables, and dairy products contain their own salt—enough, he believed, to sustain anyone who did not have to sweat in the sun to earn a day's wage. Gandhi experimented with a diet free of added salt; his example would be difficult to follow in today's world. Sodium is such a common ingredient in processed foods that salt has itself become highly processed. In the words of journalist Michael Moss, "There are powdered salts, chunked salts, salts shaped in different ways with various additives to work perfectly with processed foods." The ubiquity of salt makes it impossible for the average consumer to reduce sodium intake without a dramatic change in diet. In a society that adds salt to almost everything, sustaining a low-sodium diet entails learning how food is prepared, processed, packaged, and distributed. Gandhi modeled that kind of systematic thinking when he used the salt tax to attack colonial rule, and in his own dietary philosophy. He maintained a diet low in sodium by connecting what he ate to the larger social, political, and economic structures he strove to transform.[4]

Almost every biography of Gandhi explores the Salt March, but historians have largely overlooked its relationship to Gandhi's own dietary struggles. He may never have imagined the march had he not grappled so incessantly with salt in his daily diet. It might seem ironic for Gandhi to champion access to a substance he had spent decades avoiding. But he saw no contradiction between the Salt Satyagraha and his own efforts to limit his salt intake. By cutting salt from his own diet while attacking the salt tax, he sought health for his body and for the Indian body politic. "You can serve the country only with this body," he wrote a colleague in the run-up to his first major nonviolent campaign in India. Only with healthy bodies could nonviolent protesters achieve a healthy nation.[5]

Gandhi's embodied nationalism was far more than a banal celebration of physical fitness. To achieve true *swaraj* (self-rule), Indians had to control their land, their bodies, and their minds; this required health at every level. In Gandhi's words, "It is impossible for an unhealthy people to win *swaraj*." His expansive definition of health led him to grapple with the many obstacles to self-rule. "It is easier to conquer the entire world than to subdue the enemies in our body," he wrote. As the Salt Satyagraha made clear, achieving healthy bodies required eliminating the inequalities that kept so many Indians desperately poor. Ending poverty could not wait until after independence—it was a necessary part of independence. "To postpone social reform till after the attainment of *swaraj*," Gandhi explained, "is not to know the meaning of *swaraj*."[6]

The night before the Salt March, Gandhi scribbled a note to Jawaharlal Nehru, the future prime minister of India. "My dear Jawaharlal," he began, "It is nearing 10 p.m. now. The air is thick with the rumour that I shall be arrested during the night." If Gandhi was arrested, Nehru would need to assume a more prominent leadership role. "May God keep you," the older man wrote the younger, "and give you strength to bear the burden." Gandhi expected to be jailed long before he reached the sea. He had faith in young leaders like Nehru, but also in the common people upon whom the movement ultimately depended. If he was arrested, he declared, "let every man constitute himself into a leader."[7]

Nonviolence made such democratic leadership possible. Unlike war, civil disobedience was open to all. Anyone could manufacture, sell, or buy illegal salt. "Supposing ten men in each of the 700,000 villages in India come forward to manufacture salt and to disobey the Salt Act," Gandhi asked one crowd, what could the government do? He knew that civil disobedience would bring mass arrests and police violence. Still, the movement would continue. To struggle in the cause of justice was, like eating the right food, a vital pillar of the good life. At a prayer meeting in the days before the march, Gandhi posed a rhetorical question that laid bare the link between diet and sacrifice at the heart of the Salt Satyagraha. "What is life worth," he asked, "without trials and tribulations which are the salt of life?"[8]

Gandhi's goal was not just to change what people ate, but to transform the economic and political structures in which they lived. Through his diet, he linked questions of individual consumer choice with anticolonial social movements. As food scholar Julie Guthman has lamented, "Food politics has become a progenitor of a neoliberal anti-politics that devolves regulatory responsibility to consumers via their dietary choices." While Gandhi believed in the power of consumers, his food politics went far beyond consumer agency. Making salt affordable for the poor was one goal of his march; equally important was uniting Indians in opposition to British imperialism and ending the poverty and inequality that imperialism sustained. Would salt be enough to achieve such goals? All human beings need salt, but as Gandhi's own dietary experiments made clear, not everyone needs the same amount. Many Indians had plenty of salt regardless of the tax, and there was good reason to be skeptical that a protest focused on salt would bridge the vast divides within Indian society. Even Gandhi himself struggled to decide whether salt was a vital necessity or a dangerous temptation.[9]

FROM SALT TO *SATYAGRAHA*

The politics of salt confronted Gandhi early in life. In one of his first publications, written when he was twenty-one years old, he lamented that many poor Indians lived on "bread and salt, a heavily taxed article." In that crucial phrase, "a heavily taxed article," he made clear his disdain for the salt tax, as well as the roots of that disdain. From the beginning, concern for the poor galvanized his resistance. He published his critique of the salt tax in the *Vegetarian*, a magazine associated with the London Vegetarian Society, Gandhi's first political community. It was at a gathering of the Vegetarian Society in May 1891 that he gave his first public speech. He was "rather nervous in the beginning," but the subject of his speech—his diet—was close to his heart, and he overcame his anxiety. In his speech, he repeated the phrase "salt, a heavily taxed article."[10]

Gandhi's opposition to the salt tax grew more ferocious with time. In 1905, writing in his newspaper *Indian Opinion*, he declared that the tax "should be immediately abolished." He explained his position in terms of nutritional necessity. "Salt is an essential article in our diet," he wrote. All people need it to survive—but the poor suffered the most when the price of this basic necessity was artificially inflated. Gandhi's compassion for the poor inspired him to denounce the "injustice" of the salt tax in his book *Hind Swaraj* (Indian Self-Rule), published in 1909 and immediately banned by the British. Ten years later, he assigned a student to study the salt tax in preparation for a major civil disobedience campaign. When that campaign failed, he again decried "the blood-sucking salt tax." By depriving the Indian people of something as essential as salt, the tax revealed the profound alienation at the heart of the Raj. The question, Gandhi argued, was not just whether Indians had access to salt, but whether they had the right to self-rule.[11]

Gandhi condemned the salt tax for forty years before launching a campaign aimed at its abolition. The idea of a salt march came "like a flash" from God. The year was 1930. The New York Stock Exchange had plummeted and the world was sliding into the Great Depression. In India, economic woes galvanized the opposition to British imperialism, and Gandhi pondered how to strengthen that opposition. Targeting the salt tax provided only part of the answer. Gandhi knew he would ask protesters to gather their own salt. Should he also ask them to sell illegal salt? To march on government stores of salt? Any form of civil disobedience would be met with arrests, but marching on government property would call down the full wrath of the imperial government.[12]

Gandhi publicly debated the best form of protest. He published a letter from a retired government official who suggested restricting the movement to the collection of natural salt; taking salt from government depots "would be stealing or robbery." Using the Sanskrit word for violence, the officer stated that such a protest would be "an act of first-class *himsa*." Gandhi disagreed. He rejected the distinction between gathering natural salt from the beach and taking it from a government depot. Both forms of protest were illegal. Both were also, he insisted, legitimate forms of nonviolent resistance. "If a robber steals my grain and cooks some of it," he wrote, "I am entitled to both the raw and the cooked grain." The British had stolen salt that naturally belonged to the people of India. "The people," Gandhi argued, had "every right to take possession of what belongs to them." Convinced of the need for dramatic action, he decided to be as confrontational as possible in opposing what he called the "inhuman monopoly" on salt.[13]

Before beginning the Salt March, he wrote the Viceroy of India, Lord Irwin, in a last-minute effort at compromise. Gandhi condemned the salt tax as "burdensome on the poor man." "If you cannot see your way to deal with these evils and my letter makes no appeal to your heart," he wrote, "I shall proceed with such co-workers of the Ashram as I can take, to disregard the provisions of the salt laws." The viceroy could have him arrested, but the ultimate power resided with the people of India. If he was imprisoned, Gandhi wrote, "I hope that there will be tens of thousands ready, in a disciplined manner, to take up the work after me."

The viceroy remained unmoved. He regretted that the mahatma was "contemplating a course of action which is clearly bound to involve violation of the law and danger to the public peace." Gandhi published the viceroy's response as evidence of government rigidity, and turned to the Bible to illustrate the injustice. "On bended knees I asked for bread," he wrote, "and I have received stone instead." He used the salt tax to illustrate the absence of democracy in India. The autocratic viceroy, appointed from London, was more like a prison guard than a responsible leader; India had become "one vast prison house."[14]

To destroy that prison required the courage to confront power. The most dramatic confrontation occurred at the Dharasana Salt Works, a government-run salt factory in Gandhi's native state of Gujarat. After the completion of the Salt March, Gandhi announced that he would lead a march upon the salt works, and was promptly arrested. In his absence, he chose Abbas Tyabji, a seventy-six-year-old retired judge, to lead the protest. When the government arrested Tyabji, leadership fell to Sarojini Naidu, a renowned poet and the first female president of the Indian National Congress. Alongside Naidu marched Maulana Abul Kalam Azad, a scholar and longtime anti-imperial activist. Rather than arrest the defiant protestors yet again, the government offered a more brutal deterrent.[15]

An American reporter, Webb Miller, offered firsthand testimony of the violence that ensued. Line after line of nonviolent volunteers marched upon the salt works. Line after line, they were beaten down by the police. "Not one of the marchers even raised an arm to fend off the blows," Miller wrote. "They went down like ten-pins. From where I stood I heard the sickening whacks of the clubs on unprotected skulls. The waiting crowd of watchers groaned and sucked in their breaths in sympathetic pain at every blow. Those struck down fell sprawling, unconscious or writhing in pain with fractured skulls or broken shoulders. In two or three minutes the ground was quilted with bodies. Great patches of blood widened on their white clothes."

Miller could barely watch. "At times," he wrote, "the spectacle of unresisting men being methodically bashed into a bloody pulp sickened me so much I had to turn away." The reporter saw enough to craft a powerful narrative that he wired to newspapers throughout the world. The story appeared in over a thousand publications. American senator John Blaine read it into the official record of the United States Senate. Within India, public opinion turned even more decidedly toward independence. In the wake of the government's brutality, one Indian leader declared, "All hope of reconciling India with the British Empire is lost forever."

Not surprisingly, the viceroy took a different stance. He wrote King George, "Your Majesty can hardly fail to have read with amusement the accounts of the severe battles for the Salt Depot in Dharasana." The police, according to the viceroy, had "tried to refrain from action" but ultimately "had to resort to sterner methods." What had become an international outrage appeared to the viceroy as nothing more than a minor disturbance. He downplayed the violence of the police. "A good many people suffered minor injuries," he wrote blandly. By contrast, Webb Miller counted over three hundred injured protesters—many with severe wounds, including fractured skulls and broken bones.[16]

Gandhi had anticipated such brutality. He knew that nonviolent civil disobedience often elicits violence. In South Africa, he had seen how police atrocities attracted media coverage and galvanized further protest. In India, government repression proved similarly counterproductive. The bloodshed at Dharasana inspired sympathy from abroad and sparked a wave of protests within India. Kamaladevi Chattopadhyay, a fierce anticolonial activist and advocate of women's rights, led a protest at the Wadala Salt Works that involved some fifteen hundred protestors. Throughout India, salt was produced and sold in open violation of the law.[17]

The protests lasted nearly a year. On March 5, 1931, eleven months after the Salt March began, Gandhi climbed the stairs of the viceroy's residence to sign an agreement to end the Salt Satyagraha. It was that historic moment that prompted Winston Churchill to complain that "a seditious fakir of a type well known in the East" was "striding half-naked up the steps of the Viceregal Palace, while he is still organizing and conducting a defiant campaign of civil disobedience, to parley on equal terms with the representative of the King-Emperor." Gandhi later wrote Churchill, "I have been long trying to be a 'Fakir' and that naked—a more difficult task. I, therefore, regard the expression as a compliment though unintended."[18]

The salt protest ended with a qualified victory. The viceroy agreed to allow villagers to produce their own salt, so long as it was not for sale. The scale of the protests inspired many Indians to hope for a more radical change. For those who had sacrificed to achieve independence from British rule, a partial repeal of the salt tax seemed a paltry reward.

Despite its limitations, Gandhi celebrated the victory. Jubilantly, he encouraged volunteers to "bring the message of free salt to the semistarved villagers." He hoped villagers would produce their own salt, and expected support from the government. "At the end of our discussions," he wrote, "it became a matter of pleasure for Lord Irwin to make the concession regarding salt."[19]

Gandhi may have accurately represented the viceroy's stance. The two men had achieved some degree of personal warmth. During their conversations, Gandhi mischievously sprinkled some illegal salt into his tea as a reminder, he told the viceroy, "of the famous Boston Tea Party." The viceroy, in turn, prevented Gandhi from leaving without his shawl.

"You have not got so many clothes on," he told the mahatma, "that you can afford to leave any behind." The friendly banter masked a stubborn resistance to change. Not long after the end of the Salt Satyagraha, government officials claimed that villagers were disobeying the prohibition on the sale of salt. As a result, the right to produce salt was rescinded in many parts of India. Gandhi fought back and successfully reinstated free access to salt, but not without constant pressure from a recalcitrant government.[20]

In 1946, one year before Indian independence, Gandhi pressed the British to abolish the salt tax once and for all. "Its abolition," he wrote, would create "a feeling among the masses that the new era has already dawned." Lest colonial officials remain unmoved by the plight of the Indian masses, he appealed to British pride. "For the sake of English honour," he wrote one official, "I say that there should not be a day's delay about the abolition of this monopoly." The viceroy at the time, Lord Wavell, was not impressed by Gandhi's devotion to the cause. Privately, he deemed the mahatma a "malevolent old politician" and dismissed his concerns about the price of salt as "rather hypocritical sob-stuff." According to Wavell, Gandhi "professed to be coming purely as a friend of Britain, so that the British would get the credit of removing this unjust tax before the National Government came into power and did so." The viceroy suspected more complex motives. "The old humbug," he wrote of Gandhi, "I wonder whether he suspects that a National Government would do nothing of the sort and that the British are easier to bounce."[21]

Having failed with the British, Gandhi pressured Indian leaders to eliminate the salt tax. In the fall of 1946, he wrote to three key figures in the transitional government and offered all three the same pointed advice: "Abolish salt tax, remember Dandi March." The following day, he pressed his case at a prayer meeting in New Delhi. He reminded his listeners how many people had struggled against the salt tax. "The very first step of the Interim Government should be to abolish that tax," he concluded, "so that the poorest villager can have the feeling that the dawn of freedom has arrived."[22]

Soon after independence, the salt tax was abolished. The poor did not benefit as much as Gandhi had hoped. Inadequate distribution networks and price-gouging kept the cost of salt high. Gandhi continued to press for affordable salt for all Indians. "People say there was a time when I had marched to Dandi for salt but today there is no salt to be had or, if there is, an exorbitant price has to be paid for it," he wrote. "I can only bow down my head in shame." He encouraged poor people to make their own salt, and chided merchants and politicians for not doing more to reduce its cost. "We have become so selfish today," he declared, "that we cannot even let people have salt at a low price." British rule may have ended, but the inequality at the heart of colonialism continued to divide Indians. As he had before, Gandhi used salt to highlight that inequality. He feared that the partition of India would lead to an increased need for revenue and the return of the salt tax. "If that happens," he wrote, "too great a price will have been paid for freedom."[23]

Was a small tax on salt really too great a price for freedom? For Gandhi, freedom from British rule meant nothing if it was not freedom for India's poorest citizens. As early as 1909, he had denounced "English rule without the Englishman." The salt tax embodied the inequity of English rule. For Gandhi, a free India, by definition, had to satisfy the basic nutritional needs of all its citizens.[24]

In the method of his protest, Gandhi modeled his ideal society. Like the India of his dreams, the Salt Satyagraha was nonviolent and inclusive of diversity. Gandhi made a point of promoting religious minorities to positions of authority. Abbas Tyabji and Maulana Azad, both Muslims, were among the most prominent figures in the Salt Satyagraha. Gandhi also helped women assume leadership positions in the struggle: Kasturba Gandhi, Sarojini Naidu, and Kamaladevi Chattopadhyay were among many who took key roles in the movement. Gandhi had refused to allow women to participate in the original Salt March, citing as an excuse the gendered nature of British repression. As he told one gathering, "Just as Hindus do not harm a cow, the British do not attack women as far as possible. For Hindus it would be cowardice to take a cow to the battlefield. In the same way, it would be cowardice for us to have women accompany us." Gandhi's comparison of women and cows, like his decision to restrict the march to men, revealed the persistence of patriarchy in his philosophy and his politics.[25]

As the Salt Satyagraha swept across India, leaders like Chattopadhyay inspired Gandhi to embrace more fully the power and equality of women. Gandhi later wrote that the salt protests "brought out tens of thousands" of women "and showed that they could serve the country on equal terms with men." In 1946, he reminded his fellow Indians of the "heroism and sacrifice" of women during the civil disobedience movement. He included women and Muslims in the movement because equality was central to his vision of independent India. *Swaraj* without equality was not true *swaraj*.[26]

Gandhi defined *swaraj* through his diet as well as his politics, and the Salt March connected these concerns in ways that went well beyond the symbolic. Along the route, the marchers were fed by local residents. Gandhi made clear in advance that the food "should be the simplest possible" and that "sweets, even if prepared, will be declined." He modeled the dietary austerity he expected of his fellow marchers. "For me," he wrote, "goat's milk, if available, in the morning, at noon and at night, and raisins or dates and three lemons will do." The simplicity of his diet was an attempt to connect to India's poor; it was also a way to be a considerate guest. "I hope that the village people will incur no expenses whatever," he wrote, "except for the simple food items named above." In his attention to the marchers' menu, Gandhi demonstrated one of his fundamental beliefs: the method of any protest had to reflect the end goal.[27]

Gandhi related every aspect of the Salt March to the well-being of the body and of the nation. "The various functions in the human body have their parallel in the corporate life of society," he explained. Salt provided the most potent link between Gandhi's body and the anticolonial struggle. "The very salt I eat," he lamented, "compels my voluntary cooperation" with British imperialism. Every time he ate salt, he acquiesced in colonial rule. It was not, however, his own consumption that drove Gandhi's activism. Indeed, the greatest irony of the Salt Satyagraha is that Gandhi himself ate remarkably little salt.[28]

TOO MUCH OF A GOOD THING

Gandhi avoided salt for long stretches of his life. "As an ardent food reformer," he explained in 1930, "I have lived without any salt for over six years." His own dietary preferences did not weaken his opposition to the salt monopoly. "The way to teach people moderation in salt is not," he insisted, "to tax that otherwise most valuable commodity." He cited doctors who argued that "India's millions need more salt than they eat, and that her cattle too need much more than the poor farmers can afford to give them." Colonial taxes did not prevent the wealthy from eating too much salt, but did hurt the poor who struggled to afford their daily supply. "What is true of well-fed or overfed people," Gandhi noted, "may not be true of millions who are semi-starved and live on rice or stale unleavened cakes."[29]

How much salt is too much? In 2014, the *New England Journal of Medicine* published sharply contrasting reports on the relationship between salt and health. While one group of scientists argued that most Americans ate too much salt, another declared that the average consumer was near the *lowest* level of optimum consumption. Such debates existed in Gandhi's day as well. His response to the controversy mirrored his approach to most dietary questions: he experimented.[30]

In 1911, Gandhi's wife, Kasturba, fell ill. For one month, the couple stopped adding salt to their food. Kasturba's health underwent "a miraculous change for the better," and she decided to return to eating salt. Gandhi vowed to continue "the experiment as long as possible." For several years, he avoided any food that had been salted. "I have not yet touched the butter you gave me," he wrote a close friend. "Still on saltless diet." He knew that it was, properly understood, a low-salt diet; on a truly saltless diet, he would have died. He could survive without adding salt to his food because, as he explained, "Our diet supplies salt to us in organic forms, and that is all that we really need." After two years, Gandhi reported, "I have not come across any undesirable results from giving up salt." Indeed, he found himself more focused and energetic.[31]

Like all of his dietary adventures, Gandhi understood his low-salt diet as an effort that had to be continually reassessed in light of new evidence. He wrote a salt enthusiast to ask for proof of salt's health benefits. "If salt is the panacea for all evils," Gandhi declared, "no effort should be spared to double or even to quadruple its consumption." He never came to believe that salt was a "panacea," but he did eventually soften his opposition. Early in life, he believed that salt had "no specific utility for the body," but over time he came to accept some amount as necessary for health. "The testimony in favour of salt as a necessary article of diet is overwhelming," he wrote in 1925. Four years later, he told a correspondent, "There is no harm in taking a little salt." How much is "a little"? Gandhi told readers of his newspaper that he limited his intake to "not more than 30 grains" per day. Such precise measurement revealed his perfectionism, as well as his awareness of salt's high price for those who needed it most.[32]

Soon after he returned to India from South Africa, Gandhi witnessed firsthand the impact of the salt tax on the rural poor. In Champaran, a remote region of northeast India, he saw how the tax "artificially raised the price of salt," and made it "most difficult to procure salt at a reasonable price." To the average farmer, salt was "as necessary as water and air." Six months before he visited Champaran, Gandhi had still been on his "saltless" diet. His experience working with India's poor led him to accept salt's necessity. In a striking departure, he began to link salt to national identity, encouraging his fellow Indians to be "true to our salt, true to our nation." Salt became "the nation's vital necessity"; the poor were "the salt of India"; and nonviolent activists were "the salt of the earth."[33]

Arrested in May 1930 at the height of the Salt Satyagraha, Gandhi was sent to the notorious Yeravda prison, which he promptly dubbed Yeravda Mandir (Yeravda Temple). From his new temple, Gandhi continued to dispense dietary advice. Whereas he had previously endorsed a "saltless" diet, he now encouraged correspondents to consume salt "in reasonable quantity." He wrote, "My diet consists of three pounds of milk turned into curds and taken at two meals, and milk once. Then nine tomatoes, small or big as supplied and the required quantity of boiled vegetables such as cabbage, pumpkin, etc. I add salt afterwards if I require."[34]

A few years after the Salt March, one of his most devoted disciples decided to embark on a diet without added salt. "Abstention from salt for a time can do no harm," Gandhi wrote the disciple. Still, he cautioned against "ascribing all the good results to the absence of salt." One should not put too much faith in any dietary change. "As long as the mind is not firm and rid of passions," he asked, "how can diet alone help?" Gandhi had outgrown his dietary determinism. He still believed that moderation was crucial to physical and spiritual well-being, but moderation did not mean complete abstinence. "Salt," he concluded, "taken in small quantities can do no harm."[35]

Gandhi had always been wary of ascribing too much significance to what was eaten, as opposed to how and why it was eaten. Recall the letter he wrote his son Manilal in 1914. "Do not think that self-discipline means living on a saltless diet," the father told the son. What mattered was the meaning behind the diet. "You may live on a dry crust of bread, two days old, and a pinch of salt," he wrote. "That may, of course, be a much higher thing than my enjoying all manner of fruits and nuts." Although bread and salt were not as nutritious as fruits and nuts, the key issue was self-control. "The moral worth of our actions," he explained, "is to be judged from the motive behind your eating dry bread and my living on fruits." The moral worth came not from what was eaten but how food—or the abstention from certain foods—fueled a healthy life. Was it the challenge of a "saltless" diet that appealed to the mahatma? Was he drawn to the health benefits of abstaining from salt, or the moral benefits of absten-tion itself?[36]

Even after he developed a more balanced approach to salt, Gandhi remembered his "saltless" years as "an instance of *satyagraha*" and "one of the sweetest recollections of my life." He did not distinguish between his diet and his larger purpose; his activism shaped his diet, and his diet inspired his activism. But was that diet really *satyagraha*? Was avoiding salt the same as marching hundreds of miles to court arrest with an act of civil disobedience that shook the foundations of the British Empire?[37]

Gandhi's humility might explain why he called his saltless diet an example of *satyagraha*. Like the Salt Satyagraha, his avoidance of salt could be seen as a noble failure. "I have lived for more than forty years without condiments," he wrote in 1945, "and for nearly thirty without salt." He admitted, "It might have been a mistake on my part." Gandhi was humbled by his failures—with food as with politics. The Salt March is often remembered as a triumph of political creativity. Yet the British stayed in India for seventeen years after Gandhi led his trek to the sea. And when the Raj finally fell, the partition of India on religious lines demonstrated the limitations of Gandhi's efforts to create lasting unity. Just as the saltless diet failed to live up to its promise, the Salt Satyagraha failed to heal the divides of caste, class, religion, and gender. Gandhi rec-ognized both failures, but it was not his humility that led him to link the dietary and political dimensions of salt.[38]

Gandhi equated his low-salt diet with *satyagraha* because of the con-nections he saw between his diet and two other facets of his life: his spiri-tuality and his sexuality. He believed that salt fueled bodily passions that impeded spiritual growth. He told the business tycoon G. D. Birla, "If you give up salt and ghee for a while it will certainly help you in cooling down your passions." Going without salt could help someone achieve "a life of abstinence" vital to spiritual purity. "This saltless diet has," Gandhi told one correspondent, "materially assisted me in my *brahmacharya* vow." Often translated as "celibacy," *brahmacharya* literally means "the pursuit of Brahma," or "the pursuit of God." Gandhi believed that *brahmacharya* required "control in thought, word and action, of all the senses at all times and in all places." Achieving such sensory control required careful attention to diet.[39]

By endowing food with too much flavor, salt led to lustful eating and lustful thinking. "For controlling your mind," Gandhi wrote, "try giving up the extra salt in your food." Giving up salt fostered the self-control necessary for spiritual growth. "You can use turmeric and salt," Gandhi advised one pupil, but "a *brahmachari* should shun all these things" lest he become addicted to "the pleasure of the six flavours." The traditional Indian medical system known as ayurveda identifies six basic flavors: sweet, sour, salty, pungent, bitter, and astringent. Whereas many ayurvedic healers recommend a balance of these tastes, Gandhi was wary of the temptations of flavor and of saltiness in particular. "For everyone who wants to cultivate self-control," he offered clear advice: "Give up salt for five or six months and afterwards from time to time."[40]

Gandhi rejected any food that might tempt him to put bodily cravings above spiritual and political pursuits. Yet he struggled to distinguish dangerous pleasures from healthy delights. The mango, for example, weighed heavily on his conscience. Delicious but also nutritious, could mangoes be eaten without risking spiritual distraction? Even foods Gandhi categorically rejected had power over him—not just salt, but sugar, and the sugary treat that earned his greatest condemnation: chocolate.

CHAPTER 2

Chocolate

I see death in chocolates.

GANDHI, 1911

IT WASN'T ABOUT SATURATED FAT, LACTOSE INTOLERANCE, OR atherosclerosis. When Gandhi told a friend that he saw "death in chocolates," he was referring to the danger of passion. Few foods, he warned, were as "heating" as chocolate—heating, that is, of the fires of passion. Gandhi was a passionate man. He cared deeply about India's freedom, about nonviolence, about food. He distinguished, however, between passions. The desires of the body could distract from the yearnings of the spirit, and nothing aroused bodily desire more than the cravings of the tongue. Gluttony was not just a form of lust—it was the doorway to lust. For Gandhi, a sweet tooth was the ultimate gateway drug, weakening self-control and paving the way to a life of reckless hedonism.[1]

Consider the relationship between chocolate and sex. In the winter of 1935, Gandhi sat down with the renowned advocate of birth control Margaret Sanger. It would have been difficult to find two people who disagreed more about sex. Gandhi explained to Sanger that a couple should have sex only to produce children. "Love becomes lust," he declared, "the moment you make it a means for the satisfaction of animal needs." "It is just the same with food," he added. "If food is taken only for pleasure it is lust." As an example, he offered chocolate. "You do not take

24

chocolates for the sake of satisfying your hunger," he told Sanger. Chocolate is eaten "for pleasure." It is only for a few fleeting seconds that taste buds meet chocolate and we are given the sweet sensation of flavor. To prolong such momentary pleasures, we eat chocolate after chocolate. The result, Gandhi argued, is sickness, both physical and spiritual. As our minds turn toward chocolate, we turn away from more satisfying spiritual pleasures like prayer, meditation, and helping those in need.[2]

As with chocolate, Gandhi suggested, so with sex: the desire for bodily gratification leads to selfish and ultimately unhealthy ends, as one pleasure inflames our desire for other pleasures. Gandhi strove for "control in thought, word and action, of all the senses at all times and in all places." Chocolate and other "heating foods" complicate such control by sparking physical passion. To be safe, Gandhi recommended avoiding not only chocolate but all "heating and stimulating foods," including "condiments such as chillies, fatty and concentrated foods such as fritters, sweets and fried substances."[3]

Is eating chocolate inherently lustful? Is sex selfish? Faced with Gandhi's juxtaposition of chocolate and sex, Margaret Sanger responded, "I do not accept the analogy." Sex was not akin to sweets. Gandhi disagreed. "Of course you will not accept the analogy," he replied, "because you think this sex expression without desire for children is a need of the soul, a contention I do not endorse." Sanger retorted, "Yes, sex expression is a spiritual need and I claim that the quality of this expression is more important than the result, for the quality of the relationship is there regardless of results." In other words, sex mattered regardless of whether children were produced. Sex was an act of spiritual connection and of love. Sanger asked the mahatma, "Do you think it possible for two people who are in love, who are happy together, to regulate their sex act only once in two years?" Gandhi replied proudly, "I had the honor of doing that very thing, and I am not the only one." The advocate of birth control and the champion of celibacy found little common ground in regard to sex or chocolate.[4]

Ever since sugar became a staple of the modern diet, the consumption of sweets has been bound up with questions of virtue and vice. Part of the triangle trade that brought slaves to the Americas, sugar earned fortunes for British planters and merchants, praise from sweet-toothed consumers, and the ire of abolitionists. By creating demand for plantation labor, sugar consumption perpetuated slavery. Even after slavery was abolished, sugar plantations continued to harbor some of the worst labor conditions in the world. Desperate for cheap labor, sugar barons worked with imperial officials to bring poor Asian laborers, many from India, to work the cane fields from Trinidad to Fiji. In South Africa, Gandhi saw firsthand the desperation of indentured sugar laborers, trapped far from home in conditions not far from slavery. He decried their suffering, and explained his opposition to sugar as a response to the injustice of indenture.[5]

Gandhi denounced sweets as the product of slave labor and the source of a more intimate slavery—the slavery of sensuality. "Where there is real health," he explained, "there alone is true happiness possible, and in order to achieve real health we must conquer the palate." Disciplining desire was at the heart of Gandhi's spiritual practice. From his mother, he inherited a deep respect for Jainism, an ancient religious tradition that cherishes nonviolence and asceticism. One Jain spiritual practice involves eating bland and unappealing food known as *ayambila* in order to temper unhealthy desires. Gandhi married Jain and Hindu asceticism to a Victorian conception of self-control. If we are able to "conquer the palate," he explained, "all other organs will be automatically under our control and one who has this body under control can subdue the world because such a one becomes God's heir, a part of Him."[6]

By connecting his diet to his faith, Gandhi strove to transcend egotistical eating. Yet his extreme austerity bordered on egotism, as self-denial slipped into self-obsession. By urging austerity on his friends, family, and the general public, he enacted the polarized nature of the modern relationship with sugar. Historian Sidney Mintz has connected the rise of sugar consumption with new forms of social discipline. As people learned "to consume with more discipline," Mintz argued, morality became "a new consumable." Gandhi's dietary restraint was a form of moral consumption. His rejection of sweets was not, however, absolute. For one thing, his opposition to sweets rarely included fruit. He occasionally savored other forms of sugary treats, as well, complicating the perfectionism he brought to his diet. His occasional extravagance reveals that his love for food could, at times, trump his love for perfection—especially when the food in question was to be shared with his grandchildren.[7]

In 1940, at the age of seventy, Gandhi sent his grandson a note: "When you satisfy me with your studies . . . you are sure to find sweets in your pockets." At an interreligious meeting in South Africa in 1908, participants were served *mesul*, a sweet made with chickpea flour and coated with jelly. One speaker declared that sharing such sweets could strengthen, in Gandhi's words, "the bond between Hindus and Muslims." If candy could encourage his grandson to study, and if *mesul* could help bridge the divide between faiths, Gandhi was willing to overlook their sweetness.[8]

Gandhi associated sweets with hospitality. When a woman greeted him at a train station with "rice, coconut and a leaf-bowl of sugar-candy in her hands," he did not chastise her for the candy; he wrote an article celebrating her kindness. Travel made him grateful for culinary hospitality. In 1921, during one of his many journeys across India, he wrote his assistant from the train to ask that a few special treats be prepared for his arrival. The sweets he requested reminded him of home: *peda*, a milk sweet; *puri*, fried cakes of unleavened dough; and *golpapadi*, a dessert made from flour and unrefined sugar.[9]

Of all the delicious treats that reminded him of home, the mango would prove to be Gandhi's most lasting temptation. In his first public speech, that anxious address he gave to the London Vegetarian Society in 1891, Gandhi declared it "the most delicious fruit I have yet tasted." "Some have placed the pineapple at the top of the list," he told his audience, "but a great majority of those who have tasted the mango vote in its favor."[10]

In 1828, one English traveler described the mango as "something between a plum and an apricot." The taste was "at first, very disagreeable," but those who loved mangoes "sometimes exceed in the use of them, and prickly heat, and other disorders ensue in consequence." Mangoes did not become widely available in England until the 1970s; as late as 1931, a shipment of fresh mangoes had to be flown into London via a special flight from Egypt. Pickled mangoes were available in London at the time of Gandhi's 1891 speech, and tropical fruit of other kinds had become more commonplace. In December 1893, an Indian traveler was surprised to find fresh pineapples in the market at Covent Garden. Most likely, some members of Gandhi's audience would have traveled to lands abundant in mangoes and pineapples, and would have had their own opinions on the merits of each delicacy. Still, Gandhi spoke from a unique position of authority. He was, like the mango, an Indian import.[11]

Gandhi's mangophilia revealed more than the growing reach of imperial commodity chains. His love for mangoes demonstrated his passion for food. In 1906, after eating at a vegetarian restaurant in London, he wrote a colleague, "I had a delicious supper last night." Gandhi did not love everything he ate in England. He recoiled at bland English staples, such as the boiled potatoes and cabbage he was served at the formal dinners required of law students. By contrast, he took pride in the Indian art of cooking. In the same 1891 speech in which he lauded the mango, Gandhi noted that Indians "don't believe in plain boiled vegetables, but must have them flavored with plenty of condiments—e.g., pepper, salt, cloves, turmeric, mustard seed, and various other things for which it would be difficult to find English names unless they be those used in medicine." Ten years later, Gandhi might have cautioned against such "heating" foods. But in his twenties, he praised the "innumerable condiments" that made Indian lentil soup "a most delicious food." He even recommended a dessert made by mixing ground coconut with clarified butter and sugar. "It tastes very nice," he told his Vegetarian Society audience. "I hope some of you will try at home those coconut sweet balls, as they are called."[12]

Coconut sweet balls! It is jarring to imagine Gandhi recommending such a treat. His tastes would evolve over time. Even as a young man, his appreciation for sweets was rooted in their impact on the whole person, not just the taste buds. He recognized that delicious foods served as emotional supports. In a guide he wrote in the 1890s for other young Indians traveling to London, he suggested leaving home with "a stock of some fresh fruits and sweets," including *jalebi*, circles of deep-fried wheat soaked in sweet syrup, and *halva*, a dessert made with semolina, wheat, or carrot mixed with butter, sugar, and other spices. He also suggested that travelers bring "some salty things," offering as an example *ganthia*, a delicacy made by frying crisp small sticks of gram flour mixed with salt, black pepper, and the pungent spice *ajowan*, also known as carom seed. Gandhi made clear that students should "eat to live" rather than "live to eat." Still, his definition of "good, nutritious, healthy and palatable food" included the salty crunch of *ganthia* and a few Indian sweets to remind students of home.[13]

It was in South Africa, as he transformed himself into a social reformer, that Gandhi revolutionized his relationship to sweets. He arrived in the port of Durban in 1893, an elite lawyer who traveled first class, dressed in expensive suits, and ate the sumptuous meals expected of a gentleman of his standing. He left in 1914, a social reformer wearing Indian clothes, identifying with the poor, and having all but given up sweets. Gandhi's diet evolved as part of a total transformation in his lifestyle and identity. That transformation began in the bleak confines of a South African jail in the winter of 1908.

Later in life, Gandhi would learn to see prison as a sacred space where he could challenge unjust laws and live a simpler, more elemental existence. Such equanimity took time to develop. It was not easy for the affluent young lawyer to adjust to life behind bars. Arrested in January 1908 for defying racist laws, Gandhi launched a protest campaign to gain access to foods he would later dismiss as unhealthy luxuries. Cocoa and butter were "absolutely necessary to make bread eatable," he explained. The prison medical officer considered cocoa and butter "a relish," and had banned both from the prison diet. A more serious privation was the absence of ghee, the clarified butter common in Indian cooking. "From time immemorial," Gandhi wrote, "ghee has been considered to be the complement of rice." Those Indian prisoners who were vegetarian were given beans as a substitute for meat. "Whilst beans are an admirable substitute for meat," Gandhi declared, "they are no substitute for ghee."[14]

Gandhi would later eliminate ghee from his diet (along with cocoa and butter). In jail, he began to reconsider his attachment to particular foods. Staples he had once considered necessities came to seem more like luxuries. He criticized his fellow prisoners for their "incessant grumbling about food." They seemed to think "we lived only to eat." He focused on the need to control one's dietary desires rather than the right to satisfy those desires, and embraced an idea that was steeped in Hindu and Jain culinary traditions and that would grow in popularity in the first decades of the twentieth century—the idea that, in the words of historian Helen Zoe Veit, "self-discipline around food was a moral virtue." Such discipline was a form of gratitude, as well as a way to connect with those who had to limit their diets out of necessity. Eating in moderation, Gandhi taught his fellow prisoners, was a way to "offer thanks to God for whatever we get."[15]

Repeated stints in jail in 1908 and 1909 inspired Gandhi to empathize with the poor, and to push his diet toward the austerity forced upon millions. In the deprivations of imprisonment, he came as close to knowing poverty as an affluent lawyer could. Of course, being in prison was not the same as being impoverished. Unlike many of his fellow Indians, Gandhi did not have to worry about having enough to eat. "In India," he told readers of his newspaper, "thirty million out of a population of three hundred million get only one meal a day, and that, too, nothing more than *roti* and salt." "Compared to this," he proclaimed, "it is not much of a hardship to have to maintain oneself in gaol on three meals a day."[16]

Nothing reveals Gandhi's growing culinary compassion more than his relationship with mealie pap, a creamy corn porridge that was a breakfast staple for many black South Africans. Indians, especially middle-class Indians, tended to avoid it; racial and class prejudices combined to prevent them from eating what was widely seen as black food. Served mealie pap in jail in 1908, Gandhi rejected it. "Mealie meal is the staple of Kaffir diet," he wrote, using the pejorative term for black South Africans. "Nothing except rice," he huffed, "is acceptable to Indians."[17]

Gandhi has been justifiably criticized for drawing racial distinctions, and for failing to partner with black South Africans against white oppression. In a newspaper article on his experience in jail, he wrote, "We had fondly imagined that we would have suitable quarters apart from the Natives." He justified such segregation by declaring, "Many of the Native prisoners are only one degree removed from the animal." Gandhi's desire to physically separate from black South Africans was mirrored in his rejection of their food. His opposition to mealie pap exemplifies the racialization of diet, what food scholar Hi'ilei Julia Hobart has called "the interlocking logics of taste and territory."[18]

The boundaries of "taste and territory" were neither static nor clearly defined. For one thing, Gandhi's understanding of Indian food was decidedly diasporic—shaped by the culinary nostalgia that came with distance from India, as well as the experimentation and hybridity inspired by proximity to other culinary traditions. Moreover, his views on diet evolved dramatically during his time in South Africa, as did his views on race. These shifts in Gandhi's dietary and racial borders were related, as was made clear when he suddenly decided to embrace mealie pap after all.[19]

FROM MEALIE PAP TO CHOCOLATE

In 1899, Gandhi told the *Times of India* that "people in India would be surprised to learn that a suggestion has been seriously made that the Indians should be compelled to live on mealie (maize) meal, when the present stock of rice in the Colony is exhausted." Such a suggestion was ridiculous to Gandhi because he had already come to believe that mealie pap was not suitable for Indians. In 1908, he turned to tradition and a crude racial nutritionism to explain his opposition to the porridge. Mealie pap, he wrote, "was hardly satisfactory not because it was not palatable but because it was not a diet at all suitable for the Asiatic constitution." He accepted that Indian prisoners should eat it "if it were merely a matter of tastes," but added that "it was a matter of habit." Habit and tradition meant that Indians "could live on wheaten and rice preparations, no matter how simple they might be. But they could not live on what might be African delicacies."[20]

Gandhi's appeal to habit contradicted the radical openness he brought to most elements of his diet. Indeed, many of his dietary reforms aimed at changing outdated habits. Aware of the weakness of his position, he buttressed his opposition to mealie pap with medical arguments. In a petition to the director of prisons, he wrote that many Indian prisoners were "suffering from constipation, probably due to the eating of mealie meal." He offered no reason why the porridge would be constipating, and admitted that it did not have the same effect on all Indian prisoners. Nevertheless, he asserted that it was unhealthy for anyone with an "Asiatic constitution." He later recalled, "Even when we got over the natural repugnance, it was a diet that constipated some of us and gave diarrhoea to the others." The scattershot nature of Gandhi's critique resulted from his awareness that he lacked stronger claims and, in particular, religious grounds to oppose the porridge.[21]

In one incident, Indian prisoners suspected the dish had been cooked in lard, a travesty for vegetarian Hindus like Gandhi, and for Muslims as well. But there was nothing about mealie pap itself that was religiously taboo. Neither was its taste inherently abhorrent. "With milk, sugar or ghee," Gandhi admitted, "it can be made palatable." At stake was the relative nature of taste itself. Even while rejecting mealie pap as unsuitable for Indians, Gandhi admitted that it could be considered a "delicacy" for Africans. Such a racialization of taste could be used to police both racial and culinary borders. Yet Gandhi's growing commitment to "conquer the palate" meant that the absence of enticing flavor was, from his own perspective, a weak justification for avoiding any kind of food.[22]

In March 1908, only a few months after launching his crusade against mealie pap, Gandhi began rethinking his opposition. "Mealie pap, like wheat, is good, simple and cheap food," he wrote. "Neither can it be said to be tasteless. In fact, for some purposes, mealie pap is better than wheat." In July of the same year, he declared, "We must not imagine that eating mealie pap will do us any harm." In August, he noted that a petition had been sent by Indian prisoners asking for alternatives to the porridge, but added, "My own view is that it will be useful to accustom oneself to mealie pap."[23]

Even as Gandhi changed his views, the campaign against mealie pap found support among white South Africans. The authorities began to grant bread instead of the porridge. One white paper, the *Transvaal Leader*, endorsed Indian demands for control over their diet: "These men are political prisoners; it is unjust if they are put to hard labour or made to wear prison clothing; it is infamously unjust if they are treated dietetically as Mr. Gandhi says they are. We thought that countries professing themselves civilized had abolished torture. We seem to be an exception."[24]

It matters that Gandhi began to reconsider his opposition to mealie pap even as Indians were winning the right to eat "more suitable" foods. It was not official resistance that forced him to change his mind. Rather, the experience of jail led him to grapple anew with questions about diet, race, and class, questions that he had been grappling with for years. Although he remained focused on the rights of Indians, Gandhi had come to recognize the suffering of black South Africans and to sympathize with their struggles. He learned from several leading black South African figures, especially John Langalibalele Dube, the first president of the African National Congress. Dube had been inspired by the African American educator Booker T. Washington, and had built a rural school on Washingtonian lines. That school inspired Gandhi to create his own rural ashram focused on the Washingtonian virtues of self-reliance and the dignity of labor.[25]

In September 1905, Gandhi heard Dube speak. He reported the event in *Indian Opinion*, praised Dube's educational efforts, and declared, "This Mr. Dube is a Negro of whom one should know." When Dube became the first president of the South African Native National Congress, later renamed the African National Congress, *Indian Opinion* celebrated the new organization as an "awakening" and declared: "Our friend and neighbour, the Rev. John L. Dube, Principal of the Ohlange Native Industrial School, has received the high honour of being elected the first President of the newly-inaugurated Inter-State Native Congress." Gandhi's admiration for Dube helped drive a radical transformation of his views on race and class, a transformation that inspired his surprising embrace of mealie pap.[26]

Its humble origins became a virtue, as Gandhi came to respect the most oppressed communities in South Africa and the foods they ate. "Many Indians have a strong dislike of mealie pap," he wrote in his newspaper, "and obstinately refuse to have it." Such resistance was "an error." Gandhi called the dish "a sweet and strength-giving food," and added, "It is very tasty when sugar is added to it." In jail again in the fall of 1908, he trumpeted his enjoyment of mealie pap in an effort to set an example for his fellow prisoners. His efforts were largely unsuccessful. One of his fellow Indian political prisoners later wrote, "None of us, excluding Mr. Gandhi, who wished to show it was good food, relished it as [we did] our breakfast at home." The path of the food reformer is often lonely, but Gandhi was unfazed by the resistance to mealie pap among his fellow Indian prisoners. He savored the thick porridge even when not in jail, and served it regularly to the students at his ashram.[27]

It matters that Gandhi never fully partnered with black South Africans in opposition to apartheid, and that even when he embraced mealie pap, he did so to reform Indian society, not in order to support black South Africans struggling to regain control over their own diets, bodies, and lands. Still, Gandhi's embrace of mealie pap reveals a growing racial cosmopolitanism that would eventually inspire him to become an outspoken critic of white supremacy throughout the world. His racial cosmopolitanism became bound up with his culinary cosmopolitanism, as his growing empathy for the struggles of other nonwhite peoples found expression not only in what he ate, but also in what he refused to eat. The students who were fed mealie pap at Gandhi's ashram were not allowed tea, coffee, or hot chocolate—all of which were forbidden on grounds both nutritional and ethical. Gandhi believed that these caffeinated drinks were harmful to children; they were also "produced through the labour of men who work more or less in conditions of slavery." Gandhi would rather thirst than drink the fruits of slave labor. Fortunately, he was able to devise an alternative. "In place of these three drinks," he served "a harmless and nourishing beverage" made by steeping roasted wheat in boiling water. "Many coffee lovers cannot distinguish it from coffee," he boasted.[28]

Gandhi's wheat coffee may have been delicious, but it would not have been sweet. His ethical compass steered him away not only from tea, coffee, and cocoa, but also from sugar. By 1908, when he suggested adding sugar to mealie pap, Gandhi had already begun to wean himself from sweetness. Like the beverages he avoided, sugar was produced under barbaric conditions. On the sugar plantations of South Africa, thousands of indentured laborers, many from India, worked in conditions often compared to slavery. In 1909, Gandhi wrote, "We think that slave labour is used even in the production of sugar." His use of the phrase "we think" reveals his distance from the plight of sugar workers—as does his statement that "it is not possible to look too deeply into these matters." Still, Gandhi counseled his readers to forgo sugar, and his contact with indentured laborers increased over the course of his years in South Africa, inspired by the courage of a man named Balasundaram.[29]

In 1894, Balasundaram arrived at Gandhi's door, bloodied and beaten, with two broken teeth. His "master" had attacked him. Balasundaram had arrived in South Africa, like most Indian indentured laborers, with the hope of making a little money to bring home to his family. He found a system of harsh labor and mounting debt. Balasundaram's abusive master wielded tremendous power in a society divided sharply by race and class. As a barrister trained in London, Gandhi was one of the few Indians who could directly challenge such power. He was able to free Balasundaram, who in turn helped the affluent lawyer to confront the horrors of the labor system in South Africa. Until that point, Gandhi had evinced little concern for the poorest Indian migrants. The migrants themselves deserve credit for transforming a lawyer for the rich into a servant of the poor. "Balasundaram's case reached the ears of every indentured labourer," Gandhi wrote, "and I came to be regarded as their friend . . . a regular stream of indentured labourers began to pour into my office, and I got the best opportunity of learning their joys and sorrows."[30]

Learning the joys and sorrows of the indentured laborers was one of the greatest opportunities of Gandhi's life. That opportunity was deepened by his curiosity about the origin of his food, especially the sugar produced by workers like Balasundaram. "It is sugar made with the blood of indentured labourers," Gandhi wrote, "that we use for gratifying our palate." He linked the evils of consumption and production in a way pioneered by the abolitionists who had connected sugar to the evils of the plantation. As one abolitionist wrote in the late eighteenth century, "Every person who habitually consumes one article of West Indian produce, raised by Slaves, *is guilty of the crime of murder.*"[31]

Like the abolitionists before him and the advocates of fair trade that came after him, Gandhi aimed to uncover the moral implications of consumption chains. Even more than sugar, chocolate shaped his ethical approach to eating. Gandhi used the word "cocoa" to refer both to raw cacao beans and to the powdered cacao product we now call *cocoa*. He consumed processed cacao in the form of hard chocolate and liquid cocoa—until, that is, he rejected both. After declaring "I see death in chocolates" in 1911, he warned that there were "few substances so heating as the abominable chocolate that cursed product of devilish slave labour." In that one sentence, he connected the three foundations of his diet— nutrition, faith, and ethics. His ethical concerns reveal the geographical reach and racial inclusivity of his culinary cosmopolitanism, as cacao was neither grown in South Africa nor harvested by Indian labor. "Cocoa is produced in the Congo," Gandhi told his readers, "where indentured Kaffirs are made to work beyond all limits of endurance." In tracing chocolate to this exploitation, he demonstrated his growing compassion for the plight of black Africans. Like mealie pap, chocolate offered a dietary path to increased compassion. "In cocoa plantations," Gandhi wrote, "Negro workers are subjected to such inhuman treatment that if we witnessed it with our own eyes we would have no desire to drink cocoa." The problem was that few chocolate lovers had seen the brutality of a cacao plantation.[32]

Chocolate helped create the commodity chains that drove the great European empires. Before tea and coffee were imported into Europe, hot chocolate habituated Europeans to drinking a sweetened caffeinated beverage harvested thousands of miles away. A traditional beverage throughout much of South America, chocolate was introduced to Europe in what historian Alfred Crosby dubbed "the Columbian Exchange," the massive transfer of plants, animals, and diseases between Europe and the Americas after 1492. Not all Europeans loved the strange new American brew. The Milanese explorer Girolamo Benzoni remarked that chocolate "seemed more a drink for pigs, than a drink for humanity." A historian of chocolate, Marcy Norton, has argued that chocolate's popularity spread from the masses up the social and economic ladder. Chocolate gained popularity "from the colonized to the colonizer, from the 'barbarian' to the 'civilized,' from the degenerate 'creole' to the metropolitan Spaniard, from gentry to royalty." The taste of chocolate may have been egalitarian, but its production epitomized the inequality at the heart of colonialism, as well as the way in which commodity chains shielded consumers from direct knowledge of that inequality.[33]

Gandhi never saw a cacao plantation. He denounced the treatment of cacao workers not because of what he saw, but because of what he read. He learned to question the global supply chain of commodities by consuming an equally global flow of ideas and information. Literary scholar Pramod Nayar has written that culinary cosmopolitanism is "made possible not just by the actual availability of different varieties of food items from around the world, but also through the 'travelling' of *information, visual images, symbols* of food from round the world." Often, those symbols were created within imperial power structures that encouraged the flow of capital, people, and ideas so long as they did not threaten the status quo.[34]

As Gandhi's aversion to chocolate demonstrates, the global circulation of food information could also be turned against empire. Culinary cosmopolitanism is often assumed to mean a greater willingness to consume foods and recipes from throughout the world. Gandhi's opposition to chocolate reminds us that sometimes abstention can also be a form of transnational solidarity. Like the boycott of grapes championed by Cesar Chavez and the United Farm Workers, Gandhi's rejection of chocolate connected the ethics of abstention to an awareness of the labor conditions hidden by modern agribusiness.[35]

Gandhi never launched a boycott of chocolate. His opposition to cacao never approached his aversion to the salt tax. The production of chocolate was an abomination, but it was a distant abomination, far from his primary concerns and constituencies—whether in South Africa or in India. As with sweets more generally, Gandhi's views on cacao remained ambivalent. In South Africa, he sent lighthearted letters to the daughter of a friend, jokingly demanding that she send chocolates. In 1900, he wrote the colonial secretary to request that Indian volunteers be given the "Queen's Chocolate" that had been gifted to white soldiers who fought in the Boer War. Importantly, Gandhi did not state that he himself wanted the chocolate. Rather, he argued that it would be "prized as a treasure," a recognition of Indian service to the crown and a symbol of gratitude from the empire. Eleven years later, he would declare that he saw death in chocolates. And eight years after that, he would launch a massive campaign to free India of British rule. His opposition to chocolate—like his opposition to empire—would grow stronger with time.[36]

Gandhi recognized that many common foods were produced in ethically compromised ways. "To be sure," he wrote in 1913, "if we made searching inquiries regarding the origin of the various articles of our diet, we should feel called upon to reject 90 percent of them!" Such a realization did not lead him to apathy or despair. Rather, he focused on those foods he felt were most suspect and most easily eliminated. Sadly for chocolate lovers, "that cursed product of devilish slave labour" was at the top of his list.[37]

SWEETNESS AND SLAVERY

In July 1909, as Gandhi sailed to England to defend the freedom of Indians in South Africa, he confronted a different threat to freedom on his ship, the RMS *Kenilworth Castle*. He was no stranger to racism on public transport, having been thrown off a South African train for daring to sit in a first-class car. His anxiety on board the *Kenilworth Castle* did not, however, concern the possibility that he would be denied service because of his race or color. Rather, it was the dangers of first class that troubled him. "It is far better to be in prison," he declared, "than travel first-class on a ship." He disliked the constant attention lavished on the passengers, "looked after by servants as though they were so many babies." In a remarkable comparison, he complained, "Here I have neither the peace nor the freedom I enjoyed in gaol." In first class as in jail, he wrote, "I have to live hedged in on all sides." Unlike prison, however, luxury travel did not offer the opportunity to suffer for a higher cause. Smothered in comfort, Gandhi pined for purpose—political, personal, and spiritual. He lamented, "My prayers here lack the depth, the serenity and concentration they had when I was in gaol."[38]

Gandhi focused his reformist energies in the only direction he could—his diet. He spurned the first-class fare. "I have, as usual, two meals a day," he wrote defiantly. In addition to minimizing his meals, he also limited the kinds of food he ate. "I am growing more convinced every day," he wrote, "that I can do with still simpler food." The more he limited his diet, the more his desires decreased. He did not feel any "craving for delicacies" as he had the last time he traveled to England. He also avoided "tea and coffee as far as possible, since they are the produce of slave labour." By 1909, Gandhi had developed his critique of agricultural commodities produced by slave labor. He was also concerned with a different kind of slavery.[39]

Gandhi told his readers to avoid becoming "slaves of the palate." Locked in a cage of selfish desire, slaves of the palate lacked the compassion to live healthy lives. Constrained by ego, they became prey to personal and social maladies. At the root of "lying, pleasure-hunting, perjury, theft and so on," Gandhi found the "failure to restrain the craving of our palate." Indians fighting for freedom from racist oppression must also seek freedom from selfish desire. Anyone committed to freedom "must make a conscious effort to overcome the craving for good food that might have enslaved them."[40]

Gandhi's critique of slave labor hearkened back to the abolitionists who equated eating sugar with murder. His concerns about the slavery of the senses also had deep historical roots. In 1777, an anonymous British pamphlet attacked tea, sugar, butter, beer, white bread, and "other modern luxuries." Sugar earned special condemnation. According to the author, sugar "not only inflames the poor man's expences, but his blood and vitals also." Gandhi inherited such moral objections to sweets. He also drew upon a suspicion of flavor typical of reformers in the Victorian era. In the United States, bland food found an able champion in the prominent health promoter John Harvey Kellogg. The father of Corn Flakes, Kellogg advocated vegetarianism as well as simplicity in diet and taste. Like Gandhi, Kellogg viewed excessive flavor as a distraction from the virtues of healthy eating. "The decline of a nation commences when gourmandizing begins," he declared.[41]

Not all of Gandhi's contemporaries shared his Victorian austerity. Many Indian nationalists praised the rich flavors of Indian cooking, including the dazzling diversity of Indian sweets. Gandhi's abstention from sweets had roots in Hindu and Jain asceticism, but the consumption of sweets has long been important to many Hindu rituals. Throughout India, from temples to home shrines, many Hindus eat *prasad*, food first offered ritually to a god. *Prasad* often takes the form of sweets. Building on the connection between sweetness and prayer, the renowned reformer Swami Vivekananda used sugar to explain why a holy man would love God rather than strive to become a god. "I do not want to be sugar; I want to taste sugar," Vivekananda explained. "I want to love and enjoy the Beloved."[42]

The holiness of sweets found political significance in the resurgence of particular Hindu festivals in the late nineteenth century. The most renowned Indian nationalist before Gandhi, Bal Gangadhar Tilak, popularized a festival in honor of Ganesha, also known as Ganapati, the god whose elephant visage can be found in Hindu shrines worldwide. The festival features a variety of sweets, the most important being *modak*, a dumpling made of rice or wheat and stuffed full of grated coconut, dried fruits, and the unprocessed sugar known as jaggery. Indian sweets were too firmly established in local and regional cultures to be threatened by even the most energetic Victorian reformers. While delicacies varied from region to region, a national passion for sweets cut across divides of class, caste, and faith.[43]

Such widespread love for sweets makes Gandhi's austerity even more remarkable. Whereas the needs of the poor inspired him to moderate his resistance to salt, the relationship between sugar, slavery, and empire strengthened his aversion to sweets. His opposition hinged on the importance of self-control. His goal was not just to avoid triggers like sugar and salt, but to train the mind to be disciplined. "Merely giving up sugar, etc., will not do," he wrote. Cutting back on sweets was only one step toward "acquiring control over the mind."[44]

Discipline was for Gandhi the heart of freedom. On his way to London, he wrote about the shackles of first class. On his return journey, he wrote an even more famous tract in defense of freedom: *Hind Swaraj*, his most renowned book. As the Salt March made clear, Gandhi saw *swaraj* as much more than freedom from foreign domination. "The word *swaraj* is a sacred word," he said in 1931, "meaning self-rule and self-restraint, and not freedom from all restraint which 'independence' often means." Political *swaraj* from the British meant nothing without personal *swaraj* from the greed of consumerist society. The pathway to independence, whether for a man or a nation, was self-control.[45]

Gandhi did not entirely avoid sweets. It was "the undue prominence given to sweet things" that he worked to undermine. "Although sweet fruits supply plenty of sugar," he wrote in 1942, "there is no harm in taking one to one and a half ounces of sugar, brown or white, in the day." (This quota is roughly the amount of sugar in a can of soda, a slice of pie, or a bowl of ice cream.) Gandhi also realized that not all sugars were alike; he often contrasted brown and white sugar and described the latter as "decidedly harmful." He also distinguished between table sugar and the sugar in fruit. "Sugars are best obtained," he concluded, "from raisins, figs or dates all of which should be taken in moderation." After fruit, Gandhi preferred jaggery, known also as *gur*. "*Gur* is more nutritious than sugar," he told an audience of village-level volunteers, "because it contains salts and vitamins which sugar does not contain." In addition to jaggery, alternatives to table sugar include honey, agave, and stevia, a plant in the sunflower family often known as "sweet leaf" or "sugar leaf." Honey has an especially rich history in India, where it has been gathered wild for millennia; it is a key ingredient in many Indian desserts, including *gulab jamun*, round balls of fried dough soaked in a sweet syrup. Despite its natural origin and rich culinary traditions, Gandhi counseled moderation even with honey. For him, the ultimate goal was not to eat healthy sweets but to avoid addiction to sweets of any kind.[46]

The most important habit, Gandhi argued, is not what we eat but how much we eat. The best way to shape our sense of taste, he believed, was to eat smaller portions. "If you feel really hungry," he wrote, "I am sure you would relish salted gruel of *jowar*." What was true of *jowar*, a highly nutritious sorghum dish, was even more true of other foods. Even mealie pap tasted "quite good when one is hungry." "All the delicacies of the world," Gandhi declared, "cannot equal the relish that hunger gives to food."[47]

Relishing his meager fare, Gandhi seems an ambiguous figure. On the one hand, he found in hunger a way to savor his food without eating too much salt or sugar. But was it the food he savored, or the act of self-control? Either way, his attention was turned decidedly inward, away from the larger goals he proclaimed as the purpose of his diet. His desire for control was further complicated by the fact that he wanted more than to restrain his own palate; he wanted others to join him in his rejection of flavor. In a land in which the sharing of delicious food is one of the pillars of family and community, his austerity appears doomed.

But ascetic renunciation also runs deep in Indian history and culture. Gandhi's rejection of sugar, salt, and other spices reflected the rich ascetic traditions of a variety of Indian faiths. The spiritual grounding of his efforts to "control his palate" makes clear that those efforts were not primarily a question of nutrition, nor can they be understood as a rejection of pleasure. For one thing, Gandhi came to relish foods others would see as bland. "Taste is acquired," he insisted. After years of slowly decreasing the amount of salt in his food, for example, he found most salted foods unbearable. "Taste," he declared, "is a matter of habit."[48]

Gandhi took pleasure in renunciation itself. His asceticism is best understood as the elevation of one pleasure above another, the satisfaction of the soul rather than of the tongue. Consider, for example, his attack on chocolate as "heating." There is a rich tradition in Hindu, Jain, and Buddhist asceticism that sees renunciation itself as a heating agent—not heating of the passions, as Gandhi warned of chocolate, but heating of spiritual forces that operate in opposition to the passions. That process is known as *tapasya* or *tapascharya*, from the Sanskrit word *tapas*, which literally means "to heat." *Tapasya* is often explained as energy produced through ascetic renunciation that can burn away bad karma and thus clear the path toward spiritual advancement. If chocolate heated the passions, rejecting chocolate heated the soul.[49]

Gandhi praised *tapascharya*, and defined it as "voluntary suffering." "If we would have happiness," he declared in 1918, "we must go through suffering, do *tapascharya*." Decades later, in 1945, he defined *tapascharya* not as suffering but as "single-minded devotion," and declared,

"Whenever, in the course of my multifarious activities, I have been confronted with a difficulty of this character, this single-minded devotion has solved my difficulty in a manner which I had never expected." If *tapascharya* solves problems and leads to happiness, can it be understood as self-denial? Or would it be better to see such renunciation as self-empowerment—the replacement of cheap pleasures with a more profound and lasting freedom? In 1918, Gandhi told striking mill workers that "if our capacity for *tapascharya* or voluntary suffering is real enough, we are bound to reap the fruit." The fruit, in this case, was not self-liberation but social liberation. Gandhi's asceticism was driven by a utopian vision that reframed self-denial as the freedom not just of the individual but of the nation.[50]

SWEETS FOR THE HEART

In the winter of 1933, Gandhi sent advice to a young girl named Tangai Menon. The advice concerned the generosity of Tangai's uncle Charlie, who had, according to Gandhi, "a habit of spoiling little children by giving them too many sweets." "If I were you," Gandhi told the child, "I should distribute sweets amongst lots of poorer children and I should feel happy at the thought of sharing with them."[51]

At the heart of Gandhi's opposition to sweets was their lack of necessity. In April 1947, just a few months before India gained independence, he challenged wealthy Indians to "realize that they ought not to eat sweets and don brocades while their brethren were without food and clothing." Since they did not eat sweets to satisfy their hunger, those calories could be used better by those who needed them. "To partake of sweetmeats and other delicacies, in a country where the millions do not even get an ordinary full meal" was "equivalent to robbery."[52]

Gandhi rejected anything eaten for the sake of gratifying the palate rather than nourishing the body. Plain sugar was "an absolutely useless article of food." To be sure, the "useless" calories sugar provided were needed by many Indians; that only made the overconsumption of the rich more egregious. "Nature produces enough for our wants from day to day," Gandhi argued. "If only everybody took enough for himself and nothing more, there would be no pauperism in this world, there would be no man dying of starvation in this world."[53]

Gandhi's solution to poverty suffers from the bystander effect, the tendency for each of us to feel that our personal contribution would be insignificant. Would foregoing my evening chocolate do anything to help those dying of starvation? I could, like Tangai Menon, distribute my sweets to those in need. Or I could give money to charity rather than buying chocolate in the first place. Would the small amount of money I spend on such treats have any real impact? Why not just give money and eat my chocolate too? Gandhi's link between personal consumption and charitable giving seems unnecessary and impractical.

Gandhi recognized the many obstacles to charity. In his diet, he aimed to replace charity with what Alexis de Tocqueville called "self-interest properly understood." Avoiding sweets was not a manifestation of charity, but a way to achieve greater selflessness and thus happiness. Tangai Menon should give her sweets to the poor because they needed those calories more than she did—but also because giving would make her happy.[54]

He strove to eliminate the desire for sweets by embracing the joy of serving others. Merely craving dessert and resisting that craving would only lead to unhappiness. When some of his colleagues expressed the desire to return to legislatures they had boycotted, Gandhi wrote a trusted lieutenant that everyone should be allowed to return if that was their desire. "Those who daily attend legislatures in their thoughts should do so physically as well," he wrote. He drew an analogy with *jalebi*, the deep-fried sweet that looks like a bright orange pretzel. Molded from a fine-milled wheat flour known as *maida* and then fried, they are soaked in a sweet syrup, and sometimes flavored with rose water or lime juice. The key to perfect *jalebi* is the right combination of crisp fried dough and sweet syrup. "Is it not better," Gandhi wrote, "that one who daily eats *jalebi* in his imagination should eat the real thing and know the wisdom or folly of doing so?"[55]

Throughout his life, Gandhi wrestled with whether sweets are inherently selfish. In January 1947, as he traversed India preparing for independence, he was offered sweets by a group of women in a small town. He replied that the sweets he desired were not "for the tongue" but "for the heart." Could sweets for the tongue also be sweets for the heart? The women likely saw their gift as more than a way to please Gandhi's palate; they wanted to express gratitude, admiration, perhaps even love.

Gandhi recognized the social power of sweets as a young man in South Africa when he organized an interfaith picnic on Christmas Day. Three hundred guests were served fresh fruit, vegetables, and the rice and lentil dish known as *khichdi*. For dessert, they were given plum pudding. With age, Gandhi became more puritanical in his approach to sweets. He seemed to forget that pleasure can expand our sphere of compassion, that a good plum pudding can bring people together.[56]

Even for Gandhi, self-control was a lifelong struggle. He was not able to fully discard the desire for tasty food. "I cannot still claim," he wrote in 1913, "to have mastered the palate. . . . All that can be said about me is that I am one who is striving earnestly to attain *moksha*." Gandhi's reference to *moksha*, liberation from worldly attachments, reveals the spiritual basis of his approach to bodily desires. As revealing as his reference to *moksha* was his admission that he had failed to attain it. Gandhi's humility was at the heart of his spiritual quest. "Trying to find pleasure in food that is not particularly savoury, I ate too much today and in consequence I am ill at ease in my mind," he admitted to Jamnadas Gandhi in 1918. "If, at the age of 49 and despite this effort at discipline, I have not succeeded in bringing my palate fully under control, what may you do, in the prime of youth and living surrounded by all manner of dainties."[57]

Three years earlier, in 1915, Gandhi had pledged, along with all the members of his ashram, to control his craving for flavor. The ashram constitution declared, "Food will be simple. Chillies will be excluded altogether and generally no condiments will be used excepting salt, pepper and turmeric." Sticking to that rule was difficult, but Gandhi believed that maintaining such a vow was itself a path toward spiritual growth. "He who has his tongue under control," he wrote in 1909, "being both sparing in speech and moderate in his taste for good food, must be reckoned to have achieved a great conquest."[58]

It seems odd that an anti-imperial pacifist like Gandhi spoke so often of "control" and "conquest." Such terms appear better suited to the mouth of a Cornwallis or a Churchill. There was something distinctly imperial and at times violent about Gandhi's relationship to his body. As Parama Roy has written, "If the desire for renunciation is itself cast in terms of an inexorable drive, the relationship between violence, consumption, and nonattachment is no longer self-evident." Gandhi saw nonattachment as a form of nonviolence, but what if nonattachment required violence against the natural desires of the body?[59]

Could Gandhi conquer his own body nonviolently? Such self-overcoming was necessary, he believed, if he were to achieve freedom for himself and for his country. Indians would not be able to escape British rule if they could not transcend selfish desires. All forms of self-rule were connected to each other and to that most basic form of self-control—diet.

Gandhi cautioned against eating "dish after dish until at last we have become absolutely mad," and he blamed "the newspaper sheets which give us advertisements about these dishes" for inspiring overconsumption to the point of ill health. He lived before industrial laboratories began engineering processed foods that tempt people to eat too much, but he knew that desire was malleable; that taste and hunger were shaped, like all things dietary, by larger social, political, and economic forces. Gandhi's criticism of advertising reveals the political and economic context of his struggle to control his cravings. Conquering his body was necessary if he was to help free India, but the reverse was also true: his own bodily freedom, and the freedom of all Indians to decide their own tastes, was bound up with their collective struggle for independence. That realization helps explain Gandhi's emphasis on "control" and "conquest." In his battle against desires, more was at stake than just his own body.[60]

Both Gandhi's greatest culinary conquest and his greatest failure stemmed from his first dietary vow. As a young man, he promised God that he would not eat meat. He remained vegetarian for the rest of his life, but his understanding of vegetarianism was neither simple nor static. He struggled to attain sufficient protein and experimented with a variety of sources—including eggs and dairy. Being vegetarian challenged his idealism, stretched his creativity, and ended in what he saw as one of the greatest tragedies of his life.

CHAPTER 3

Goat Meat and Peanut Milk

Behold the mighty Englishman,
He rules the Indian small
Because being a meat-eater,
He is five cubits tall.

A RHYME GANDHI LEARNED IN HIS YOUTH

GANDHI WAS BORN INTO A VEGETARIAN FAMILY, BUT AS A TEENAGER came to believe that meat would allow him to grow stronger. If thousands of Englishmen had conquered millions of Indians, the meat-fueled strength of the British must be to blame. Indians would have to alter their diet if they were to gain their freedom. One day, young Gandhi secretly tried a few bites of goat. "Tough as leather," the first few chunks left him disgusted. That night, he had a recurring nightmare. "Every time I dropped off to sleep," he recalled, "it would seem as though a live goat were bleating inside me, and I would jump up full of remorse."[1]

His remorse was not enough to prevent him from continuing the experiment. In small doses, over the course of a year, he secretly played the carnivore. Eventually, his shame at lying to his parents convinced him to return to vegetarianism. It was only later, as a student in London, that he developed his own reasons to avoid meat, and what had been mere custom became the foundation of his identity. "A bloodless diet should prove very beneficial in every way," he concluded in 1895, at the age of twenty-six. He praised vegetarianism for "its immeasurable superiority to flesh foods on grounds scientific, sanitary, economic, ethical and spiritual." His meatless diet helped connect his most important beliefs about ethics, politics, and physical and spiritual health. At the heart of those connections, a core idea began to emerge, an idea that would come to define him as a world figure: nonviolence. More than any other facet of his life, Gandhi's vegetarianism inspired his devotion to nonviolence, to *ahimsa*. More than a political tactic, *ahimsa* was a religious commitment to the dignity of all beings.[2]

As his commitment to vegetarianism deepened, Gandhi grappled with whether he should also forgo eggs and milk. Ultimately, he became convinced that he should become vegan, and renounced all animal products. Living without eggs was relatively easy. Doing without milk, by contrast, proved to be one of the greatest challenges of his life. He experimented with almond milk, peanut milk, and other vegan alternatives. In 1914, he vowed to abstain from all dairy products. But after contracting a serious illness, he decided that his pledge did not include goat's milk.[3]

Is it wrong to eat meat? Does drinking milk harm the planet? Gandhi grappled with the nutritional, ethical, and political consequences of consuming animal products. A steadfast vegetarian but a failed vegan, he defied many of the stale binaries that cloud discussions of how we use animals for food. From goat meat to goat's milk, Gandhi's winding path fostered a tolerance for difference that would prove central to his nonviolence. But his deep regret at his failed veganism prevented him from being fully tolerant with himself.[4]

THE PERFECT WAY

Gandhi believed the human body was designed to run on plants. "The structure of the body," he wrote in 1913, "would seem to indicate that Nature intended man to be a vegetarian." Thirty years later, he repeated his belief that vegetarianism was especially suited to human physiology. "His teeth, his stomach, intestines, etc.," he wrote, "seem to prove that nature has meant man to be a vegetarian." The key word in both of these pronouncements is "seem." The human body only *seemed* to prove that vegetarianism was the most natural way. Despite his firm beliefs, Gandhi respected other views on the relationship between meat and health. He acknowledged that many doctors believed eating meat was healthy.

"Medical opinion," he wrote, "is mostly in favour of mixed diet." Even as he held firm to his own vegetarian principles, he remained open to being wrong.[5]

Most of Gandhi's vegetarian colleagues were far less humble. Anna Kingsford, one of the first English women to receive a medical degree, authored a best-selling defense of vegetarianism in 1895. Its title was revealingly confident: *The Perfect Way in Diet*. Kingsford argued that the shape and function of the human skull, teeth, and stomach proved that the human body was designed to run on fruits and vegetables. She linked meat to illness and, in turn, argued that vegetarianism could cure many ailments.[6]

Gandhi repeatedly told audiences that a vegetarian diet had freed Kingsford of tuberculosis. In South Africa, he sold copies of Kingsford's book, and offered to pay the advertising costs himself, in order to spread the gospel. Like Kingsford, Gandhi believed in the nutritional benefits of a vegetarian diet. Unlike Kingsford, he harbored doubts as to whether vegetarianism was "the perfect way" for all people. His balanced approach contrasts sharply with the polemical one-sidedness that often divides the "experts" on both sides of today's vegetarian debate.[7]

Despite his deep faith in vegetarianism, Gandhi worried about whether his diet provided sufficient nutrition. Those worries grew stronger when he stopped drinking milk. In 1918, he wrote one of his sons that it was "difficult, without the use of fats and what they call proteins, to rebuild a body grown weak because of the vow not to take milk." The phrase "what they call proteins" reveals that the word had not yet become commonplace. Over the course of the 1920s, the necessity of protein became widely accepted, and Gandhi began using the term regularly. When one South Indian doctor promoted a diet of banana and coconut milk, Gandhi challenged the doctor on nutritional grounds. "Is it not a fact that banana and coconut contain little or no protein," he wrote, "whereas, milk contains comparatively a fair amount of protein?" Gandhi wished that bananas provided more protein; they were a staple of his diet, and he struggled with his dependence on milk. Still, he refused to place wishful thinking above science.[8]

In Gandhi's day, most Western doctors believed that the more protein one ate, the better. This myth played an important role in the pseudo-scientific discourse that underpinned the British Raj. In 1912, a colonial official named David McCay authored a seminal work that used comparisons between "the different tribes and races of India" to argue that higher amounts of protein led to "a high development of physique and manly qualities" while its absence resulted in "poor physique, and a cringing effeminate disposition." Of course, the meat-eating British were amply supplied with protein and "manly qualities."[9]

Gandhi confronted the colonial preference for meat head-on during a public debate with British India's closest thing to a food czar. The director of nutrition research for the government of India, Sir Robert McCarrison, was a towering figure in nutritional studies and the author of a "food primer" aimed for Indian children. Gandhi approved of the book, but criticized its focus on the necessity of meat and milk. Despite the work of scientists like McCarrison, Gandhi declared, "The unlimited capacity of the plant world to sustain man at his highest is a region yet unexplored by modern medical science."[10]

McCarrison replied in a cordial but challenging letter. He praised Gandhi for approaching his dietary experiments with "open-mindedness," but suggested that the mahatma was wrong about the capacity of the plant world to provide complete sustenance. Science, he wrote, had made clear "the nutritive limitations of a purely vegetable diet." In contrast to Gandhi's vegetarian optimism, McCarrison asserted, "Man's digestive tube is not long enough nor capacious enough to accommodate a sufficient mass of suitable vegetable food." Gandhi published McCarrison's letter, but refused to cede the medical higher ground to meat eaters. He assured readers, "There are medical men who are decidedly of opinion that animal food including milk is not necessary for sustaining the human system to the full." Scientists had only begun to investigate "the hidden possibilities of the innumerable seeds, leaves and fruits for giving the fullest possible nutrition to mankind." The paucity of scientific research on the potential of a vegetarian diet was not accidental. Gandhi decried "the tremendous vested interests that have grown around the belief in animal food." Such vested interests prevented doctors "from approaching the question with complete detachment."[11]

Gandhi's concerns remain relevant at a time when food companies fund studies that boost the health claims of their products, and the meat and dairy industries pour money into advertising. *Milk has calcium that is good for your bones. Meat has protein that will make you strong.* Backed by industry-funded research, such messages influence doctors as well as the general public. Unlike in Gandhi's era, however, today's medical establishment has become much less committed to meat. While most doctors would dispute Gandhi's belief that the body was designed for vegetarianism, the vast majority would also reject McCarrison's claim that the human digestive system requires animal products. Too many healthy vegans prove otherwise. Medical opinion has embraced the healthfulness of vegetarian and vegan diets. Gandhi reached the same conclusion more than one hundred years ago. "Muscular vegetarians," he declared in 1896, "demonstrate the superiority of their diet by pointing out that the peasantry of the world are practically vegetarians, and that the strongest and most useful animal, the horse, is a vegetarian, while the most ferocious and practically useless animal, the lion, is a carnivore."[12]

Gandhi cared about the nutritional impact of meat and dairy, but he recognized that health concerns alone offer a weak foundation for vegetarianism. For one thing, meat eaters can be perfectly healthy. "Health," he acknowledged in 1931, was "by no means the monopoly of vegetarians." Conversely, rejecting meat does not guarantee health. Gandhi lamented that many vegetarians "made food a fetish" and "thought that by becoming vegetarians they could eat as much lentils, haricot beans, and cheese as they liked." Being a vegetarian should not be an excuse for gluttony. Gandhi criticized fellow vegetarians for "talking of nothing but food and nothing but disease." Instead, vegetarians should develop "a moral basis" and "an altruistic purpose." A single-minded focus on health could inhibit altruism by directing attention toward the body and away from the most important end of a vegetarian life—the happiness of other living beings.[13]

PORRIDGE AND PIE

Gandhi believed that eating meat involves "the infliction of unnecessary pain on and cruelty towards harmless animals." By avoiding such cruelty, vegetarianism opened a path toward transcendence of the self in service of other living beings. Like refusing chocolate, rejecting meat was more than a negative act; it was an affirmation of spiritual values. From his childhood, Gandhi's vegetarianism was rooted in religious systems that valued all living beings. Jains strive toward complete nonviolence; some wear masks to avoid inhaling insects. Within Hinduism, vegetarianism has equally deep roots, and not just for Brahmins. Many devotees of Vishnu, known as Vaishnavas or Vaishnavites, are also vegetarian. Gandhi was born into a Vaishnavite family with strong ties to Jainism. His vegetarianism was doubly blessed.[14]

Before crossing the "dark water" to England, Gandhi promised his mother that he would avoid "wine, women, and meat." Although given in the presence of a Jain priest, Gandhi's vow did not protect him from being ostracized by some members of his caste. Many Indians remained convinced that England was a land of pollution and sin. Some of Gandhi's friends warned him that he would never survive the brutal winter without eating meat. One English doctor told him that "in the cold climate of England the addition of beef or mutton is essential." The doctor sternly declared, "You must either take beef-tea or die!" Gandhi responded, "If it were God's will that I should die I must die, but I was sure it could not be God's will that I should break the oath that I made on my mother's knee before I left India."[15]

It was not easy to keep that oath. Gandhi's first four months in England were a culinary catastrophe. Bland boiled vegetables could not match the spicy delights of India. As a student, Gandhi was required to attend a series of formal dinners at his law college. Students ate family style. A group of four received a slab of meat, usually either beef or mutton, as well as some fruit and two bottles of wine. Gandhi abstained from the meat and traded his wine for extra fruit. But he could not survive on fruit alone. Day after day of bread, fruit, and bland vegetables left him weak in body and spirit.

Salvation came in the form of a vegetarian restaurant. "The sight of it," Gandhi remembered, "filled me with the same joy that a child feels on getting a thing after its own heart." He would never forget his "first hearty meal" since arriving in London. "God had come to my aid," he later explained. Divine providence took the form of English oats, as Gandhi ate porridge for the first time. "I did not at first enjoy it," he remembered, "but I liked the pie which I had for the second course."[16]

In the company of fellow vegetarians, Gandhi found more than delicious food; he found a new identity. His introduction to the world of British vegetarianism was simultaneously physical and intellectual. Before he entered the vegetarian restaurant, he had spotted a series of books for sale in a small window, and purchased one of them, Henry Salt's *Plea for Vegetarianism*. Salt was the intellectual godfather of the British vegetarian movement. Born in India, the son of a British army officer, he had developed a dietary faith just as deep and devoted as the religious conviction of Gandhi's family. Salt's philosophy sprang from an ethical ideal that encompassed all living beings. "It is not human life only that is lovable and sacred," he wrote, "but all innocent and beautiful life: the great republic of the future will not confine its beneficence to man." After reading Salt, Gandhi recalled, "I adopted vegetarianism from principle."[17]

Salt was only one of many British vegetarians to have a strong influence on Gandhi. London was a meat-eating city, but also a thriving hub for vegetarians, many of whom were even more zealous living amidst so many carnivores. With the passion of a marginalized minority, vegetarians built a network that aimed to support their own while attracting new converts. In Gandhi, they found the ideal recruit. Although long committed to vegetarianism as a practice, he was new to vegetarianism as a movement. Once he had found a reason to reject meat, he did so with the fervor of the recently converted.

Vegetarianism was at the center of an entirely new way of living. London's vegetarians tended to oppose industrialization, urbanization, and war, and to support non-Western and nontraditional spiritual traditions. Unlike in India, British vegetarianism had emerged on the fringe of established society. The term *vegetarian* entered the English language in the 1840s. In 1847, a Vegetarian Society was founded in Manchester. Its membership drew primarily from two earlier organizations: the Bible Christian Church, a religious community led by a visionary vegetarian pastor, and the Alcott House Academy, an alternative school, named after Bronson Alcott, father of the novelist Louisa May Alcott. In 1888, the London Vegetarian Society was formed. It would play a major role in shaping Gandhi's vegetarianism and his political activism more generally.[18]

Vegetarians in Victorian Britain were simultaneously backward-looking and forward-looking. They saw abstaining from meat as part of a larger shift in lifestyle, radical in its break with society but conservative in its vision of returning to an unspoiled past. The renowned poet Percy Bysshe Shelley epitomized the movement's romantic utopianism. According to Shelley, "abstinence from animal food" would allow "the advantages of intellect and civilization" to be "reconciled with the liberty and pure pleasures of natural life." Gandhi repeatedly included Shelley in lists of famous vegetarians, but his strongest ties were with the vegetarians he befriended during his time in London.[19]

Gandhi's closest vegetarian friend was Josiah Oldfield. A barrister with an Oxford pedigree, Oldfield could have lived a comfortable life as a lawyer. Instead, he pursued a medical degree and edited the journal of the London Vegetarian Society. Perhaps his most radical decision involved his living situation: he decided to share a home with a young, impecunious student from India named Mohandas Gandhi. Oldfield and Gandhi lived together in a quiet house overlooking a leafy park, just a mile's walk from London's Paddington Station. The two men often entertained other vegetarians. Their parties featured rice, lentil soup, and dried fruit. As a provincial Gujarati student—shy and socially conservative—the young Gandhi might have seemed an unlikely host for gatherings of English radicals. But vegetarianism allowed him to explore new identities while remaining comfortably anchored on familiar ground. It helped that so many of London's vegetarians were respectful of Hinduism and other non-Western religions. Gandhi rightly saw, in the words of scholar Leela Gandhi, the "zoophilia of his English companions as a variety of xenophilia: that openness to outsiders, aliens, strangers, foreigners."[20]

In England, Hinduism had long been associated with vegetarianism. Anna Kingsford called Hindus one of "the first civilised communities." Amongst them, she wrote, "a pure vegetable diet is regarded as the first essential of sanctity." Kingsford and Gandhi were drawn to Esoteric Christianity, a hodgepodge of Christian and "Oriental" mysticism that appealed to many of London's vegetarians. In South Africa, Gandhi would publicly identify himself as the "agent for the Esoteric Christian Union and the London Vegetarian Society." Not all of London's vegetarians were so religiously ecumenical. Arnold Hills, a pious man with strong ties to the Congregationalist Church, described vegetarianism as "a moral force whose momentum shall overthrow the kingdom of darkness." Gandhi called him "a puritan." Despite their differences, Hills and Gandhi became close colleagues. Faith inspired both men's vegetarianism.[21]

Most of Gandhi's vegetarian friends understood their dietary habits as ethical choices. They strove to live healthy lives, but their diets were guided just as much by consideration for other living beings. Gandhi found such kindness toward animals a revelation, especially in the capital of imperial Britain. "May I say in all humility," he told Henry Salt, "that one rarely finds people outside India recognizing non-human beings as fellow beings." Gandhi praised Salt for recognizing the "grand truth" that all animals deserved compassion. Gandhi strove to put that truth into practice. He told his older brother, "My family now comprises all living beings."[22]

Gandhi believed that vegetarianism could foster a healthier, more just world for all animals. Like most of his contemporaries, however, he neglected what has since become one of the most powerful arguments in favor of abstaining from meat—that it is better for the planet. The production of a vegetarian diet—fruits, vegetables, nuts, grains—requires fewer resources than meat. Gandhi saw that disparity in economic terms: at a hotel in London, he recalled with dismay that the bill for a single meal came to more than a British pound, a large sum at that time. At a vegetarian restaurant, by contrast, he purchased a full meal for a bit more than a shilling, nearly twenty times cheaper than the carnivorous alternative. "Vegetarian foods are the cheapest diet," he concluded. The economics of a meat-free diet offered hope for the poor. Vegetarianism could, Gandhi predicted, help end "the rapidly growing pauperism" that went "side by side with the rapid march of the materialistic civilization and the accumulation of immense riches in the hands of a few." Such grand pronouncements reveal Gandhi's utopian streak. He overlooked the fact that vast numbers of India's poor were already vegetarian, often by necessity. A vegetarian world would use natural resources more efficiently, but the challenge of fair distribution would remain. If vegetarianism was to end poverty, it would have to end greed first.[23]

Gandhi believed vegetarianism could abolish greed by replacing sensual egotism with spiritual compassion. He overstated his case when he claimed that "religious teachers of all the religions" agreed "that nothing is more detrimental to the spiritual faculty of man than the gross feeding on flesh." Many religious teachers eat meat. When Martin Luther King visited India, and was asked whether his conception of nonviolence included vegetarianism, he responded with one word: "No." Gandhi was not, however, alone in linking vegetarianism and spirituality. By emphasizing abstention and austerity, he connected his vegetarianism to multiple faith traditions.[24]

Gandhi's spiritual objection to meat dovetailed with his desire to control his palate. Rejecting meat could, he believed, free anyone from the constraints of selfishness and ego. He went so far as to claim that vegetarianism was "the safest and surest cure for drunkenness." Little evidence links meat-eating and alcoholism, but for Gandhi the two were connected forms of slavery to the body. "All those who suffer from the craving for drink," he concluded, "have only to give a trial for at least one month to a diet chiefly consisting of brown bread and oranges or grapes, to secure an entire freedom from the craving." Freedom from craving, freedom from desire—that was the independence, the *swaraj*, Gandhi most prized. Like the British Empire, meat and wine deprived the individual of that most basic right—the freedom to be at peace with oneself. "The most ardent vegetarians," Gandhi noted with approval, "attribute the agnosticism, the materialism, and the religious indifference of the present age to too much flesh-eating and wine-drinking, and the consequent disappearance, partial or total, of the spiritual faculty in man." Without that "spiritual faculty," no one could claim the autonomy necessary to live free of addiction.[25]

Autonomy was much more than a personal goal for Gandhi. If his freedom depended on an ethical diet, so did the freedom of India. This was the self-rule that Gandhi would seek with the Salt March, with his rejection of sweets, and again with his vegetarianism. He knew that it was not enough for him to change his own diet; social justice requires social action. Gandhi believed that his dietary changes reinforced his activism, and his activism fueled his diet. Nothing reveals that symbiosis more than his vegetarian politics. Gandhi arrived in London a painfully shy young man, terrified of speaking in public, and left a committed activist, with new confidence as a writer and a public speaker. Vegetarianism helped turn a quiet student into a confident leader. Sociologist Lauren Corman has written of "the ventriloquist's burden" that confronts animal rights advocates and all those who aspire to speak on behalf of the voiceless. Too often, self-proclaimed advocates have misrepresented the needs of those they claimed to defend. What does it say about Gandhi that speaking on behalf of others gave him his own voice?[26]

Vegetarian activism taught Gandhi two vital skills for a budding political leader—networking and fundraising. He learned both from Arnold Hills. The man Gandhi had called "a puritan" was also one of the most powerful vegetarians in London. The managing director of the Thames Iron Works, a shipbuilding company, Hills bankrolled the London Vegetarian Society and its newspaper, the *Vegetarian*. He envisioned vegetarianism as an international movement and launched the Vegetarian Federal Union, an effort to connect vegetarians throughout the world. Gandhi learned of the union at a meeting of the London Vegetarian Society in Portsmouth, a bustling town located on the island of Portsea, off the southern coast of England. A report on the union was read aloud, its purpose stated in grand terms: "Our aim is a bold, and ambitious one, to bind together in one harmonious whole, the disciples of Vegetarianism; to concentrate their efforts, to strengthen their hands when needed; and this not within the bounds of our own seas, but the four quarters of the globe."[27]

The internationalism of the Vegetarian Federal Union inspired Gandhi's own global vision. As a first step toward world unity, he hoped that vegetarianism could heal the rift between Britain and India. Writing in the *Vegetarian Messenger* in 1891, he envisioned a time "when the great difference now existing between the food habits of meat-eating in England and grain-eating in India will disappear." Rather than Indians becoming more like the British by eating meat, he hoped that the British would become more like Indians by avoiding meat. Such a culinary shift might inspire the "sympathy that ought to exist between the two countries." Gandhi's emphasis on sympathy reveals his political thinking at the time, more cautious reformism than radical anti-imperialism. At least vegetarianism allowed him to invert the prevailing power dynamic that assumed all civilized things flowed from Britain to its colonies.[28]

The vegetarian community pushed Gandhi to find his own voice, and to have the courage to speak his mind. Elected to the executive committee of the Vegetarian Society, he attended every meeting but never spoke. "I always felt tongue-tied," he later wrote. Oldfield, his friend and housemate, challenged him: "You talk to me quite all right, but why is it that you never open your lips at a committee meeting?" In his autobiography, Gandhi explained, "I was at a loss to know how to express myself. All the rest of the members appeared to me to be better informed than I. Then it often happened that just when I had mustered up courage to speak, a fresh subject would be started. This went on for a long time." Invited to speak at a public meeting to promote the cause of vegetarianism, he wrote his speech in advance, but had to have a friend read it. He was too shy to read his own words.[29]

Gandhi's reticence was challenged when a controversy divided the London Vegetarian Society. The group counted among its founding members Thomas Richard (T. R.) Allinson, a doctor who advocated for vegetarianism as well as other controversial reform efforts, including birth control. Like Gandhi, Allinson served on the society's executive committee. Allinson's public support for birth control made him a divisive figure, and conservative members such as Arnold Hills mobilized against him. As Gandhi remembered it, Hills "thought that the Vegetarian Society had for its object not only dietetic but also moral reform, and that a man of Dr. Allinson's anti-puritanic views should not be allowed to remain in the Society." Gandhi was torn. He saw Allinson's support for birth control as "dangerous," but he nevertheless "thought it was quite improper to exclude a man from a vegetarian society simply because he refused to regard puritan morals as one of the objects of the Society." The stated purpose of the group "was simply the promotion of vegetarianism and not of any system of morality." Gandhi believed "that any vegetarian could be a member of the Society irrespective of his views on other morals." He wanted to share his opinion with the other members of the executive committee, but he was afraid to speak, and so wrote out his opinion in advance. "So far as I recollect, I did not find myself equal even to reading it, and the President had it read by someone else," he recalled. Despite this intervention, Allinson was expelled. Gandhi's efforts were not without meaning, however. He would maintain a connection to Allinson in the years ahead, and the experience of taking a public stand on a controversial issue forced him to confront his shyness.[30]

Slowly, he found the courage to speak in public. In the summer of 1891, he attended a meeting of the Band of Mercy, an animal rights organization. When the scheduled speaker fell ill, Gandhi was asked to take her place. He agreed, and despite his fear of public speaking, delivered a fifteen-minute lecture "on vegetarianism from a humanitarian standpoint." Later that summer, he left England, having completed his studies. On June 11, the *Vegetarian* reported his farewell speech to the vegetarians who had become his family away from home. The newspaper described the speech as "very graceful though somewhat nervous." The fact that Gandhi rose and spoke, despite his nerves, demonstrates the confidence he had gained through his participation in vegetarian politics. According to the newspaper, all in attendance believed that Gandhi was going to do "still greater work for vegetarianism." He did not disappoint.[31]

In South Africa, Gandhi continued to champion the cause. As in London, many of his closest friends and colleagues were vegetarians. He frequented the Alexandra Tea Room, Johannesburg's only vegetarian restaurant. One of his closest friends, Albert West, offered a vivid portrait of the restaurant and its clientele: "Around a large table sat a mixed company of men comprising a stockbroker from the United States who operated on the Exchange in gold and diamond shares, an accountant from Natal, a machinery agent, a young Jewish member of the Theosophical Society, a working tailor from Russia, Gandhi the lawyer, and me a printer." That young Jewish theosophist might have been Henry Polak, one of Gandhi's most intimate friends. Polak was as passionate about vegetarianism as Gandhi. After the two men bonded over their shared love for onions, Polak suggested they form an "Amalgamated Society of Onion-Eaters."[32]

Gandhi's vegetarianism yielded new friends and a new community, a precious gift in a society that was increasingly inhospitable to anyone without white skin. But rejecting meat could also strain friendships. In Durban, Gandhi befriended a white couple, the Askews, who took to hosting the young lawyer for dinner every Sunday. During one of those dinners, Gandhi decided to offer a lesson on vegetarianism to the youngest Askew, a five-year-old boy. "I spoke derisively of the piece of meat on his plate and in high praise of the apple on mine," Gandhi remembered. "The innocent boy was carried away," he recalled, "and joined in my praise of the fruit." When Gandhi returned the following week, he learned that the boy had been asking for fruit instead of meat all week long. Mrs. Askew was not pleased. "If he gives up meat," she worried, "he is bound to get weak, if not ill." Henceforth, she asked that Gandhi avoid discussing food with the child. Gandhi sagely noted that his actions would speak louder than words. If Mrs. Askew was worried about her son becoming vegetarian, it would be best if Gandhi stopped coming for dinner. She agreed, he remembered, "with evident relief."[33]

Despite the occasional run-in with a carnivorous mother, Gandhi's vegetarianism enriched his social life. The practice of abstaining from meat spanned nations, religions, and cultures. Indeed, Gandhi's vegetarianism challenged the very idea of distinct cultures by bridging his Gujarati Vaishnavite upbringing and the world of genteel British society. In his vegetarianism, as in so many facets of his diet, Gandhi rejected the divide between East and West. He envisioned a global crusade against meat-eating: "If some men of means, and well up in vegetarian literature, were to travel in different parts of the world, explore the resources of the different countries, report upon their possibilities from a vegetarian standpoint, and invite vegetarians to migrate to those countries which they may consider suitable for vegetarian propaganda, and, at the same time, worth settling in from a pecuniary point of view, much vegetarian work can be done, openings can be found for poor vegetarians, and real centres of vegetarianism can be established in various parts of the world." Gandhi's vegetarianism was radical in its zeal and its global scale.[34]

From India to Britain to South Africa, Gandhi traversed an increasingly interconnected world, and his vision for a global vegetarian revolution mirrored his mobile lifestyle. Meanwhile, many American vegetarians were becoming more insular and less political. In the words of historian Adam Shprintzen, "From 1817 until 1921, movement vegetarianism shifted its aims from conquering social ills and injustice to building personal strength and success in a newly individualistic, consumption-driven economy." Gandhi's vegetarianism appears even more radical when placed in comparison to such a trend. If he had moved to America rather than South Africa, his vegetarianism might have narrowed along with his politics. As it happened, Gandhi's vegetarianism grew more radical with time—radical in its links to utopian politics and anticolonial activism, and radical in the depth of what it demanded of the individual vegetarian.[35]

Imagine a few vegetarians stranded in the Arctic. Faced with a choice between eating meat and starvation, what should they do? Gandhi posed that thought experiment in 1921. A true vegetarian, he concluded, "will meet death but not eat meat." "That alone is *dharma*," he explained, "which is followed at the cost of one's life; anything else is mere convenience or amusement." *Dharma*, sometimes translated as "religion" or "faith," was for the mahatma a spiritual duty that connected the individual to a larger sacred order. Vegetarianism linked Gandhi's identity to his *dharma*. He could not eat meat and remain himself. Such an adamant stance on vegetarianism makes it even more striking that Gandhi was tolerant of those who did eat meat.[36]

TOLERANCE AS *AHIMSA*

In 1894, soon after his arrival in South Africa, Gandhi sent a circular letter to the Indian community he had left behind in England. He pleaded with his fellow Indian expatriates to take decisive action on behalf of India—not by denouncing British rule, but by joining the vegetarian movement. Gandhi envisioned vegetarianism as a bridge spanning the divide between India and Britain. "The vegetarian movement will indirectly aid India politically," he wrote, "inasmuch as the English vegetarians will more readily sympathize with the Indian aspirations." Such a vegetarian anti-imperialism was, Gandhi assured his readers, validated by his own "personal experience." He had found many British vegetarians to be especially sympathetic to India's cause, and encouraged his fellow vegetarians to "come forward" to "prove that Britain and India can be indissolubly united by the chain of love." That hopeful idea neglected not only the fact that the vast majority of Britons ate meat, but that a large number of Indians did as well.[37]

More than any other country in the world, India evokes vegetarianism. Yet the majority of Indians eat meat. Gandhi knew that vegetarianism was a divisive issue; whether to eat meat and which meat to eat—these questions separated Hindu from Muslim, high-caste from low-caste. Early in life, Gandhi declared vegetarianism "a movement every Indian should have at heart." With time, he came to realize the divisiveness of that goal. "It is futile," he told a colleague in 1924, "to think that under the swaraj of the immediate future everyone will become a vegetarian." Gandhi's vegetarianism did not trump his other core values. To a colleague struggling to care for the poor and the sick, he did not hesitate to suggest meat as an option. "To meat eaters you may unhesitatingly give meat-soup," he wrote. "This is not the time for doing our religious duty of propagating vegetarianism."[38]

In pursuit of India's unity, Gandhi was willing to accept those who ate meat. His tolerance was inspired by his British vegetarian friends. Henry Salt, for example, famously defended gradualism as the most practical path toward his vegetarian utopia. Gandhi's tolerance also stemmed from his own struggles with vegetarianism. Long after his childhood experiment with goat meat, he continued to agonize over the limits of his vegetarianism. Part of the problem was that the meaning of "vegetarian" varied greatly. Many Indian vegetarians refused eggs. "They argue," Gandhi explained, "that to eat an egg is equivalent to killing life." Most Indian vegetarians did, however, consume milk and butter. By contrast, some of the "vegetarian extremists" he encountered in London rejected all animal products, including dairy. Writing in the *Vegetarian* in 1891, Gandhi left unsaid his doubts about dairy, perhaps because they had not yet fully formed. On the question of eggs, he was more forthright, if a bit sheepish. He admitted, in parentheses, "(I am sorry to say I have been taking eggs for about a month and half.)" By recognizing that his actions were not perfect, Gandhi revealed the humility at the heart of his vegetarianism.[39]

Humility is the only logical response to the roller coaster that is nutritional science—a series of contradictions nowhere more confusing than in the case of eggs. During Gandhi's lifetime, the egg was heralded as an inexpensive source of protein. After cholesterol became linked to heart disease in the 1950s and 1960s, the egg plunged in popularity, at least among health-conscious consumers. Recently, the egg has been embraced yet again, as decades of studies have failed to offer solid proof that dietary cholesterol influences blood cholesterol. Freed from the specter of heart disease, eggs now appear to be a low-cost form of high-quality protein, packed with omega-3 fats, choline, and a range of other nutrients. For Gandhi, whether to eat eggs hinged on a single question: should the egg be considered a living being? As with many facets of his diet, Gandhi approached that question with flexibility. In 1891, he ate eggs, albeit apologetically. By 1909, he was avoiding not only eggs but also products that contained eggs, even the free pudding served on board the ship he took to London. In 1927, he considered eating unfertilized eggs, which were "as much without life and therefore unobjectionable as milk." In some ways, eggs were even better than milk; as Gandhi explained in 1930, by eating unfertilized eggs "we do not deprive any creature of its food, as we do by taking milk." Gandhi believed that eggs would complicate his efforts at celibacy and self-restraint, and thus continued to avoid them, but no longer because of his vegetarianism. He continued to worry about the pain that hens felt when caged, but was willing to grant that "it may be necessary in some cases to recommend innocuous eggs as medicine."[40]

Gandhi's flexibility with eggs mirrored the tolerance he extended to meat-eaters. In a remarkable conversation he shared in 1940 with a group of anticolonial activists, he was asked, "Should one stop with the human species or extend *ahimsa* to all creation?" He responded carefully: "For the Congress *ahimsa* is naturally confined to the political field and therefore only to the human species." His interlocutors pushed him: "Then what about meat-eating and egg-eating? Are they consistent with nonviolence?" "They are," he replied firmly. "Otherwise we should have to exclude Mussalmans and Christians and a vast number of Hindus as possible coworkers in *ahimsa*." Forced to choose between human unity and vegetarianism, Gandhi did not hesitate to prioritize humanity. Although his own conception of nonviolence included vegetarianism, he refused to treat his own beliefs as universal. "I have known many meat-eaters to be far more nonviolent than vegetarians," he concluded.[41]

Gandhi's approach to dietary *ahimsa* also reflected his humor. In Yeravda jail in 1932, he often began his day by drinking hot water with honey and lime juice. He would allow the steaming liquid to cool for a few minutes before taking his first sip. One day, he placed a piece of cloth over his glass. One of his colleagues, Vallabhbhai Patel, assumed that Gandhi was, like the Jains he admired, trying to avoid killing tiny organisms. Patel commented, "We cannot observe *ahimsa* to such an extent." Gandhi laughed and replied, "We may not observe *ahimsa* but we must see that our food and drink are free from dirt." Such a willingness to subtly mock his most important commitments helped Gandhi avoid the polarizing divisions that marked vegetarianism in his day, as in our own.[42]

In Gandhi's India, no issue was more divisive than the killing of cows. Gandhi was still a child when a cow protection movement spread across India. Beef-eating tended to map onto religious lines, and the protection of cows often pitted Hindus against Muslims. Championed by the Hindu revivalist organization, the Arya Samaj, the movement took a violent turn in the 1880s. Riots targeted Muslims accused of slaughtering cows. Conflict over cow slaughter has continued to plague India, as armed mobs have attacked and killed Muslims, Dalits, and others accused of killing, eating, or otherwise harming cows.[43]

Gandhi firmly opposed the killing of cows. "Even meat-eaters," he declared, "should abstain from beef-eating." At stake was more than a sacred animal. Gandhi believed that caring for cows could inspire a broader compassion for "the entire sub-human world." Despite his devotion to the cow, however, Gandhi denounced the use of cow protection to demonize Muslims, and rejected the use of violence to protect cows. "The only method I know of protecting the cow," he wrote, "is that I should approach my Mahomedan brother and urge him for the sake of the country to join me in protecting her." His commitment to nonviolence inspired tolerance toward those who ate beef. "It is not religion, but want of it," he declared, "to kill a Muslim brother in order to save a cow." Rather than violence, "courtesy" and *satyagraha* should be used to convince beef eaters to change their ways.[44]

Gandhi never initiated *satyagraha* on behalf of India's cows. Instead, he focused on "courtesy" as the path to protection. After dining at the home of a Muslim friend, he published an account of the meal in his newspaper. Although his Muslim friend was not a vegetarian, Gandhi did not "catch even a glimpse of meat in his house." "Because of his observing such decorum," he wrote, "our friendship was strengthened, not weakened." Rather than attempt to convert his friend to vegetarianism, Gandhi celebrated how the two men could get along despite their differences.[45]

His commitment to tolerance did not prevent Gandhi from challenging his nonvegetarian friends to debate the ethics of their diet. In 1920, he wrote a meat-eating colleague about "the broad humanitarian ground" involved in vegetarianism. "I consider that God has not created lower forms of animal life for man to use them as he will," he explained. All living beings deserved respect as part of God's creation. "I have no right to destroy animal life," he argued, "if I can subsist healthily on vegetable life."[46]

While Gandhi used reason to appeal to nonvegetarians, others invoked his name to support more coercive tactics. He publicly denounced activists who claimed that he "had prohibited the use of meat to any Hindus or Mussulmans," and lamented the fact that "meat and fish were even forcibly taken away from people by over-zealous vegetarians." Such violent vegetarianism was anathema to the mahatma. "It is generally known that I am a staunch vegetarian and food reformer," he acknowledged. "But it is not equally generally known that ahimsa extends as much to human beings as to lower animals and that I freely associate with meat-eaters." All living beings deserved to be treated with *ahimsa*. "It is violence, not nonviolence," he made clear, "to prevent someone from eating the kind of food he likes to eat."[47]

Gandhi believed meat-eating was harmful. He distinguished, however, between degrees of harm. "Some violence is unavoidable," he explained. "Even plants have life," and we cannot entirely avoid injuring them. "We eat vegetables," he wrote, "and yet do not think that we commit violence in doing so." Eating meat was more violent than eating vegetables—but attacking your neighbor because he ate meat was an even more egregious form of violence.[48]

Gandhi's expansive nonviolence was shaped by fellow vegetarians like Henry Salt, who was a pacifist, and Josiah Oldfield, who founded the Society for the Abolition of Capital Punishment. Before Gandhi gained world attention, the most famous vegetarian proponent of nonviolence had been the Russian novelist and social reformer Leo Tolstoy. Eating meat, Tolstoy wrote, was "simply immoral, as it involves the performance of an act which is contrary to moral feeling—killing." Tolstoy's belief in nonviolence went far beyond matters of diet. In his nonfiction magnum opus, *The Kingdom of God Is Within You*, Tolstoy argued that war is incompatible with "a religion founded on peace and goodwill toward men." Gandhi was "overwhelmed" by "the independent thinking, profound morality, and the truthfulness" of Tolstoy's book. In a speech in September 1928, he used explicitly religious language to credit Tolstoy with inspiring his nonviolence. "When I went to England," Gandhi declared, "I was a votary of violence, I had faith in it and none in nonviolence." After reading Tolstoy, "that lack of faith in nonviolence vanished."[49]

Gandhi's faith in nonviolence kept him from eating meat, and prevented him from attacking those who did eat meat. As with salt and chocolate, he believed that whether someone ate meat was not as important as how she lived her life. From a spiritual perspective, vegetarianism should not be seen as "an end in itself." As he put it, "Many a man eating meat but living in the fear of God is nearer his freedom than a man religiously abstaining from meat and many other things, but blaspheming God in every one of his acts." Gandhi's tolerance for nonvegetarians also stemmed from his self-perceived failure as a vegetarian, a failure that came in the form of milk. "I have given very deep thought to the subject of milk," he wrote in 1915. "It is objectionable from so many points of view that it ought to be avoided altogether." He experimented with veganism "times without number," but ultimately decided he needed milk to thrive. He deemed his failure to avoid milk "the tragedy of my life." Confronting that tragedy helped him learn to tolerate the failings of others, even if he was never able to forgive himself.[50]

PEANUT MILK

Arrested for defying the salt tax in May 1930, Gandhi was imprisoned in Yeravda jail. In an effort to publicize their benevolence as well as Gandhi's peculiarities, the British government paraded before reporters "a dozen wooly animals of the purest strain, purchased by His Majesty's Government to supply the prisoner with his favourite beverage: goat's milk." By the 1930s, Gandhi was drinking goat's milk regularly; it was a gross error, however, to call it his "favourite beverage." He came to goat's milk reluctantly and with considerable regret.[51]

Gandhi's opposition to milk was a "matter of ethical principle" steeped in the profound importance of the cow within Hindu tradition. As historian Kendra Smith-Howard has written, "To take milk's history seriously is to understand the compromises, complexity, and challenges involved in our dependence on other organisms for our very sustenance." That dependence was especially complicated in a religious context in which cows were venerated. In Gandhi's opinion, cow's milk was "but another form of meat and man has no right to take it." What he called the "moral drawback" of milk consumption began with his compassion for cows, but extended to more intimate concerns.[52]

Gandhi believed that milk weakened his ability to remain chaste. "Giving up milk and milk products helps one in observing *brahmacharya*," he explained in 1925. His views were shaped by an influential spiritual teacher, a Jain jeweler named Raychand, who linked milk to sexual libido. Many Hindus, by contrast, saw milk as an especially pure and "cooling" liquid that posed no risk to spiritual transcendence. Rejecting convention, Gandhi became convinced that milk threatened *brahmacharya* and thus spiritual progress.[53]

For six years, from 1912 to 1918, he refused all dairy products. His resolve was shaken during a trip to London in 1914: in bed with a severe illness, he found himself weak and in pain. When his doctors advised milk in order to strengthen his body, he "flatly refused," explaining that he had "vowed not to consume it and would not therefore have it" even if he "should die without it." Unlike his concerns about salt, Gandhi's opposition to milk stood on a religious foundation. "I have taken a final vow here not to have milk and ghee," he explained. "I will never consume these things in this present life."[54]

Gandhi stuck to his vow and recovered. He received help from T. R. Allinson, the vegetarian doctor he had supported despite their differing views on birth control. Instead of dairy products, Allinson advised brown bread, raw vegetables, fresh fruit, oil massages, regular walks outdoors, and keeping the windows open day and night. Gandhi liked "all these suggestions," but it is unclear how helpful they were for his health. The treatment "thoroughly overhauled me," he recalled, "but did not completely cure me." Still, Allinson provided expert justification for Gandhi's belief that "the cure lay not in taking medicine internally but in dietetic changes assisted by external remedies." Perhaps most importantly, Allinson reassured Gandhi that he did not need milk.[55]

Gandhi encouraged others to take up a dairy-free diet. He was not convinced the diet would work for everyone; although several children in his school had given up milk without "ill effects on their health," he worried about depriving growing children of nutrition. He continued to keep dairy out of his own diet, however, and strove to convince others to do likewise. His housemate in Johannesburg, Millie Polak, had agreed to forgo sugar (because it was produced by indentured labor) and onions (because they "heated" the passions). But she remained firm when it came to dairy products. If milk was so harmful, she asked, why was it given to children? "A man shall be judged by what comes out of his mouth," she told Gandhi, "not what by what he puts in it." Gandhi granted that milk could be healthy for children, but reiterated his opposition to milk for adults. His arguments proved unpersuasive, and milk continued to flow within the walls of the Gandhi-Polak residence, even if Gandhi himself refused to drink it.[56]

It was in 1918, in the midst of the First World War, that Gandhi returned to drinking milk. When a severe bout of dysentery reduced him "to a skeleton," doctors advised dairy. At first, Gandhi refused. As his health continued to deteriorate, his wife and his doctor worked together to convince him to consider his state of mind when he vowed to never drink milk. Was he thinking only of cow's milk? If so, why should the vow prevent him from drinking goat's milk? After some prodding, Gandhi relented to this artful logic and took up a glass of goat's milk. "It seemed to bring me new life," he remembered.[57]

Goat's milk may have strengthened Gandhi's body, but it weighed heavily on his soul. "Truly speaking," he wrote, "for one who has given up milk, though at the time of taking the vow only the cow and the buffalo were in mind, milk should be taboo." Throughout the remainder of his life, Gandhi lamented his dependence on goat's milk. He abhorred what he called his "slavery to milk," but remained convinced he needed it to have the strength to fight British imperialism. "If I were not working in public life," he explained, "I would again give up milk and continue my experiment." The physical demands of the anticolonial struggle required that milk remain in his diet—or so Gandhi thought.[58]

During his vegan years, he believed not only that milk was unnecessary for health, but that it often weakened his health. After his bout with dysentery, however, he became convinced that "in order to keep perfectly fit, vegetarian diet must include milk and milk products such as curds, butter, ghee, etc." His change of heart seems baffling given the abundant evidence that a vegan diet can be perfectly nutritious. Gandhi lived before the dairy industry launched a massive campaign to sell milk as a vital source of nutrients; calcium, in particular, has been presented as uniquely available in dairy. Many vegetables provide calcium, and it is unlikely that Gandhi needed dairy to get enough calcium. His concern was more likely with protein. He often avoided beans and lentils because of difficulty with indigestion. Without meat, dairy, beans, or lentils, he may have found it difficult to consume sufficient protein.[59]

Gandhi remained hopeful that he could be healthy without dairy—if only he could find the right substitute. "I am convinced," he wrote, "that in the vast vegetable kingdom there must be some kind" of alternative "which, while supplying those necessary substances which we derive from milk and meat, is free from their drawbacks, ethical and other." That was in 1942, almost twenty-five years after he had begun drinking goat's milk. For decades, Gandhi strove to find a replacement for dairy. In the midst of his struggle with dysentery, he asked an eminent chemist for "an exact vegetable substitute for ghee and milk." He inquired about milk made from "delicate *mhoura* seed." (The *mhoura* plant, from the genus *Bassia*, never lived up to Gandhi's hopes. Its cousin, *Bassia scoparia*, by contrast, has become renowned for its seeds, which are known as "land caviar" and eaten with delight in Japan and China.) Gandhi also looked in more conventional directions: he produced his own coconut milk and praised olive oil as "a good substitute for milk in many ways."[60]

Gandhi's greatest hope came in the form of almond milk. He loved nuts, and almonds in particular. As early as 1891, in one of his first published articles, he declared, "Almonds are supposed to be very good for the brain." One of Gandhi's arguments with his wife reveals the importance he attached to nuts. After he admitted an untouchable family into his ashram, Kasturba protested. Although she supported many of her husband's social reforms, Kasturba harbored conservative views on caste. In order to overcome her resistance, Gandhi took drastic measures: he gave up nuts. By eliminating such a vital pillar of his diet, he aimed to demonstrate the depth of his emotion. "I had to undertake partial starvation," he later explained. His nut fast succeeded in overcoming his wife's belief in untouchability. The tactic demonstrated Gandhi's stubborn adherence to what he believed was right, as well as the centrality of nuts to his diet.[61]

By 1913, Gandhi had developed his own homemade almond milk. He recommended "a preparation of sweet almonds made by soaking them in hot water, peeling and grinding them to a fine paste and mixing this thoroughly with water." Such almond milk had "all the beneficial properties of milk and none of its risks." Over time, he realized that the skin had nutritive value and stopped peeling his almonds. Instead, they were "wiped with a clean dry piece of cloth and pounded fine along with the skin." In addition to almond milk, he also experimented with making almond paste and almond jelly. To make his almond jelly, he soaked the nuts in hot water until the peel was easily removed. He then crushed the peeled almonds into a paste and mixed the paste with a small amount of water. Finally, he boiled the result until the water evaporated and a "butter-like jelly" was left behind. He ate his almond jelly with vegetables. Although his primary focus was on the nutritional and ethical benefits of replacing cow's milk with almond milk, he was not unconcerned with the taste of his creation. "One can add a little jaggery or sugar," he advised, "or even lime juice and salt to the liquid."[62]

While he perfected his almond milk, Gandhi received a recipe from George Washington Carver. Famous throughout the world for his experiments with peanuts, Carver had developed a peanut milk that Gandhi hoped might become his panacea. The peanut had come to India from the Americas, and now Gandhi turned to an African American scientist to reimagine its use. Carver believed his peanut milk helped the mahatma. Speaking before the governor of Mississippi in 1937, Carver announced that he was aiding Gandhi in his struggle against the British. Several newspapers reported the claim: "The eminent chemist, born of slave parents in Missouri, and who as a child was stolen and traded for a race horse, also revealed that the lowly Alabama peanut, not the Indian goat, furnishes Mahatma Gandhi with the remarkable strength he possesses." The newspapers stated that Carver's peanut milk had become "constantly included" in the mahatma's diet. Gandhi praised Carver as a genius, published an article about him in India, and sent several notes to him through colleagues. Gandhi's papers do not indicate, however, whether he found Carver's recipe helpful. If he did drink Carver's peanut milk, it did not eliminate his need for goat's milk. Neither did almond milk. Gandhi offered varying explanations for the failure of nut milks. The cost and availability of nuts may have played a role. Indigestion was also a challenge. The fats from nuts were, he told one correspondent, "too strong for my delicate stomach."[63]

In the search for a lasting solution to his most distressing dietary problem, Gandhi welcomed advice. Lady Cecilia Roberts, a British aristocrat with a generous heart, suggested malted milk. A mixture of malted barley, wheat flour, and cow's milk, malted milk often came in the form of a powder whose health benefits were widely touted. The malting process, in which the barley is allowed to germinate, produces a sweet richness that gives malted drinks their distinctive flavor. Unfortunately, Lady Roberts overlooked the fact that malted milk contains cow's milk. After researching the substance and discovering its bovine origins,

Gandhi politely wrote Lady Roberts "and asked to be relieved from having to take it." Gandhi was aware of his own dietary peculiarity, and did not want his diet to cause offense; he knew that his vow to avoid milk might be misunderstood. After summarizing his interactions with Lady Roberts in a letter to a close friend, he added, "The fact is I look upon life as one of discipline and restraints. These things are often caricatured as in the tortures that the so-called yogis go through. But in their essence they will stand the closest scrutiny."[64]

Although he continued to avoid cow's milk, Gandhi stopped advising friends to abstain from dairy. "I see that it is useful for preserving one's life and health," he explained in 1925, "and, therefore, no longer advise anyone to give it up." As he had with salt, he recognized that milk served an important function in the life of India's poor. He called milk of "paramount value to the nation," and encouraged women to abjure foreign clothes and invest instead in buying "milk and ghee for your children." In 1947, a few months before India gained independence, Gandhi helped distribute powdered milk to the children of poor Muslim refugees. "Powdered milk does not have the vitamins fresh milk has," he wrote, "but the inherent nutritive property of milk is preserved in powdered milk." His concern for India's malnourished children led Gandhi to endorse milk's virtues. In an article on children's health, the same man who had lived without dairy for six years declared, "More than anything else, milk is a perfect food."[65]

During his dairy-free years, Gandhi saw milk as a mother cow's gift to its child, and used the sanctity of breast-feeding to argue for veganism. "We are certainly not entitled to any other milk except the mother's milk in our infancy," he argued. As he embraced the necessity of milk, his speeches and writings filled with references to the importance of mother's milk as a source of physical and spiritual sustenance. The breast-feeding mother became the epitome of life-giving sustenance. "I cling to India like a child to its mother's breast," he wrote in 1921, "because I feel that she gives me the spiritual nourishment I need." It wasn't just India that was akin to a nursing mother. Gandhi used the analogy to explain his early commitment to the British Empire and his later attachment to the Indian National Congress. The Gujarati language also became a mother figure: "I must cling to my mother tongue as to my mother's breast, in spite of its shortcomings. It alone can give me the life-giving milk." In a remarkable discourse on kindness, Gandhi directly compared the human mother and the mother cow as beneficent givers of milk. He asked: "And what is that fellow-feeling without the milk of human kindness? Do you feel anything like the love that a cow feels for her calf or a mother for her baby? The cow's udders and the mother's breast overflow with milk at the sight of their young ones. Do your hearts overflow with love at the sight of your famished countrymen?"[66]

In New Delhi in 1947, not long before he was killed, Gandhi used the breast-feeding mother as an analogy for the interreligious harmony he hoped would come to India. At one of his prayer meetings, he declared: "A child feeds at his mother's breast because it is his duty to do so. And this alone gives him the right to live. This is a paramount law and no one can change it. If Hindus consider Muslims their brothers and treat them well, Muslims too will return friendship for friendship."[67]

None of the above examples involve Gandhi directly encouraging the human consumption of cow's milk. Even his comparison between the human mother and the lactating cow could be used as an argument for veganism. It was, after all, the sight of the calf that inspired the cow's udders to "overflow with milk." While all of these analogies could be employed in defense of veganism, Gandhi did not use them that way. Instead, his praise for mother's milk coincided with his shift toward an embrace of cow's milk as a public good.

Even as he celebrated milk, Gandhi continued to lament its necessity in his own diet. In his newspaper, he reprinted a note from Sir Robert McCarrison, the same doctor who had lectured him on the necessity of meat. McCarrison staunchly defended the importance of milk. He argued that "the greatest nutritional need of India" was "the freer use of good milk." Milk would be good for Gandhi too, McCarrison suggested in a personal postscript. "When next you make an Andhra tour," he told the mahatma, "avoid 'the extreme weakness' which overtook you in your last one, by taking a pint of milk a day!" Responding to McCarrison's letter in the pages of his newspaper, Gandhi reassured the doctor, "There is no danger of my decrying milk until I have obtained overwhelming evidence in support of a milkless diet." "By instinct and upbringing I personally favour a purely vegetarian diet," he wrote, "and have for years been experimenting in finding a suitable vegetarian combination." Until he found that "vegetarian combination," he would continue to drink goat's milk and to promote cow's milk for the Indian masses. "It is one of the many inconsistencies of my life," he explained, "that whilst I am in my own person avoiding milk, I am conducting a model dairy which is already producing cow's milk that can successfully compete with any such milk produced in India in purity and fat content." His public support for cow's milk and his reluctant consumption of goat's milk both stemmed from the same fundamental principle: food should fuel public service. He praised milk because it provided needed nutrients for the poor. He drank goat's milk because he believed it was the only thing that could give him the strength to fight for *swaraj*.[68]

Utopian but also deeply considered, Gandhi's passionate vegetarianism and his lapsed veganism both reveal how nonviolence connected his diet, his politics, and his faith. As his flexible vegetarianism makes evident, his nonviolence was built on a foundation of tolerance and humility. His open-minded understanding of vegetarianism grew directly from his own frustration with the challenge of eating ethically. He first confronted that challenge as a teenage vegetarian in a society in which eating meat was associated with modernity, progress, and power. But it was milk that drove home for Gandhi that even he could not achieve the perfect diet. If the purpose of his diet was to transform the world, milk taught him to pursue that goal humbly and tolerantly. Any other way would be a form of violence.

Many students of Gandhian nonviolence have noted its fundamentally transnational and cross-cultural roots. It is not just that Gandhi studied in London or that he was inspired by figures like Thoreau and Tolstoy. His conception of nonviolence was rooted in a spiritual quest that he saw as profoundly universal. In the words of Thomas Merton, "Gandhi's dedicated struggle for Indian freedom and his insistence on non-violent means in the struggle—both resulted from his new understanding of India and of himself after his contact with a *universally valid* spiritual tradition which he saw to be common to both East and West." Gandhi's culinary cosmopolitanism laid the foundation for his nonviolence, not just by leading him to connect his vegetarianism to a larger critique of inequality and injustice, but also by inspiring him to see in vegetarianism a way to link the personal and the political, the nutritional and the spiritual. As Merton wrote, "The whole Gandhian concept of non-violent action and *satyagraha* is incomprehensible if it is thought to be a means of achieving unity rather than as *the fruit of inner unity already achieved.*" Gandhi's diet linked such inner unity to the global solidarity he sought through *satyagraha*.[69]

Gandhi revealed the purpose of his diet in an exchange with the wealthy Indian industrialist G. D. Birla. After making a fortune in the jute business and expanding into textiles, tea, and motor vehicles, Birla decided to use some of his wealth to support the cause of India's freedom. He asked Gandhi how to be of service. Gandhi responded by ordering Birla to eat more yogurt. "Take curds without fail," he instructed. Yogurt would help keep Birla healthy and thus more able to serve his country. It remains unclear what Birla made of Gandhi's connection between diet, health, and service, but it must not have troubled the industrialist too much. He went on to become one of Gandhi's most important supporters and one of India's most renowned philanthropists. He would have many opportunities to receive dietary advice from the mahatma, as would most figures in Indian politics. Gandhi would become known as a dietary maverick and something of an eccentric. His struggle with dairy was peculiar in a society that prized milk. But his efforts to become vegan were less strange than his suspicion of cooking itself. In India, where the arts of the kitchen are treasured, Gandhi's experiments with raw food constituted one of his most revolutionary ventures.[70]

CHAPTER 4

Raw, Whole, Real

It is out of our ignorance that we believe we get our bread because
of our efforts. It is best if one realizes that He who has given us
teeth will also give us food for chewing.

GANDHI, 1909

FOR TWELVE DAYS IN THE SUMMER OF 1893, GANDHI ATE NOTHING
but raw food. This was not his first experiment with what he called
"vital food," nor would it be his last. Later in life, he would go months
without cooking his food. What makes those twelve days in 1893
remarkable is that he kept a food diary in which he carefully recorded
everything he ate and everything he felt. He had arrived in South Africa
only a few months earlier, a twenty-four-year-old lawyer from India
thrown into a profoundly racialized society. He had been kicked off a
train for daring to ride first class and had been physically abused by a racist stagecoach driver. Perhaps it was the shock of his new world and its
racist inequalities that inspired the young Gandhi to focus on something
he could control: his diet.[1]

The first entry of Gandhi's raw food diary, dated August 22, 1893:
"Began the vital food experiment. . . . Had two tablespoonfuls of wheat,
one of peas, one of rice, two of sultanas, about twenty small nuts, two
oranges, and a cup of cocoa for breakfast." The last item is telling. Gandhi
had not yet rejected chocolate as "that cursed product of devilish slave
labour." More significant at the time was the way in which he prepared his carefully planned meal. He soaked the wheat, peas, and rice

overnight, but did not cook them. It took him forty-five minutes to eat the meal that left him feeling "very bright in the morning." By evening, however, he experienced "depression" and "a slight headache." The next day brought more unpleasant symptoms: "Feeling hungry, had some peas last evening. Owing to that I did not sleep well, and woke up with a bad taste in the mouth in the morning." On the third day, he "woke up uneasy, with a heavy stomach." The heaviness lingered, as he suffered a persistent indigestion that lasted into the fifth day of his trial. "The vital food," he concluded, "does not seem to agree well."

Always reluctant to end an experiment, Gandhi soldiered into the second week of his raw diet. For a moment, it seemed he might turn a corner. "Woke up well in the morning," he reported on day seven. For breakfast, he had an orange, twenty nuts, one and a half tablespoons of wheat, and two tablespoons of sultanas. For dinner, he ate "three tablespoonfuls of wheat, two of currants and twenty nuts and two oranges." Finally, in the evening, he ate "some rice, vermicelli and potatoes." Gandhi's diet was limited by the scarcity of fruits and vegetables, and by his frugality. His experiment might have gone more smoothly if he had access to avocados and other staples of raw food diets. Whether a result of his choices or of his constraints, his raw food diet was not going well. "Felt weak towards evening," he jotted down in his diary.

On September 2, twelve days after abandoning cooked food, Gandhi returned to his usual diet. He delighted in "porridge, bread, butter, jam and cocoa." Eating "the old food" left him feeling "ever so much better." He did not, however, reject raw food categorically. Like a scientist, he never saw a particular experiment as the last word on a subject. Although his trial had failed, he declared, "Vital food may have its grand possibilities in store." Gandhi would continue to experiment with raw food throughout this life. Although he never permanently abandoned cooked food, his experiments with uncooked food grew more successful over time.[2]

Raw food appealed to him for many reasons. Chief among them was its simplicity. "That I could dispense with cooking, that I could carry about my own food wherever I went, that I should not have to put up with any uncleanness of the landlady or those who supplied me with food"—all of these reasons led Gandhi to praise the "extreme simplicity" of a raw diet. He also offered nutritional justifications. Like many advocates of a raw diet, he believed that nutrients could be lost in the process of cooking. He expressed special concern for the vitamin A "in leafy vegetables and germinated grains of cereals." "Green leaves, tomatoes or cabbage must be taken uncooked," he wrote. "Vitamin A is destroyed by the mere applying of heat." In order to boost vitamin intake, he noted, "many people take raw vegetables, pulses, wheat, etc., which have sprouted after being soaked in water."[3]

Gandhi saw uncooked food as a way to cleanse the body and the world of impurities. His belief in the social power of raw food places him in opposition to the many philosophers and scientists who have asserted that cooking distinguishes human beings from other animals. The Scottish writer Samuel Johnson put it succinctly: "My definition of man is a cooking animal." The French anthropologist Claude Lévi-Strauss used the dichotomy between "the raw and the cooked" to distinguish between nature and culture. More recently, the British primatologist Richard Wrangham has argued that cooking played a decisive role in human evolution. Raw food enthusiasts tend to reject the divide between humanity and other animals. Gandhi's turn toward the raw reflected his ecological awareness that people cannot be separated from nature. But his raw diet was not a rejection of civilization. Instead of equating cooking with civilization, he believed that raw food could make humanity more civilized.[4]

VITAL VEGETABLES

Deathly ill in London in 1914, Gandhi was prescribed milk by his doctors, but decided to try a different change in his diet. "Even in this dangerous condition," he wrote a relative, "I am making experiments." He described his dietary experiment as follows: "In the morning, I have soup with two or three teaspoonfuls of dry banana . . . and ground-nut, with tomatoes and a spoonful of oil added. At noon, I take a small carrot and one half of a small raw turnip, with eight biscuits, made of wheat or banana flour, boiled. Sometimes, in place of carrot and turnip, I take two leaves of cabbage, crushed. In the evening, two spoonfuls of rice, boiled, with vegetables as above or dry figs, soaked in water, with a small piece of bread made of banana flour or wheat." Three things about Gandhi's London diet deserve attention. First, he ate primarily fruits, vegetables, and nuts. Second, he was partial to the banana, a fruit unjustly maligned because of its relatively large number of calories (about one hundred), despite its rich amounts of potassium, magnesium, and fiber. Gandhi relished banana bread, banana biscuits, and banana soup. During one of his trips to London, his ship ran out of ripe bananas. He arranged for the crew to bake half-ripe bananas. "Among fruits," he stated, "bananas occupy the first place."[5]

The third key facet of Gandhi's London diet is more subtle but even more important. He ate much of his food raw. He boiled his rice, cooked his biscuits, and most likely warmed his banana, peanut, and tomato soup. But much of his daily diet—his carrots, turnips, cabbage, and figs— he ate raw. In this moderate experiment with raw food, Gandhi offered an unusually balanced approach. Take those banana biscuits, for example. He started with green bananas, peeled and cut into thin discs. He placed these banana chips in the sun for three days. Once they had become "quite dry and brittle," the banana chips could be stored for future use, eaten, or cooked. "With nuts and oil and tomatoes," Gandhi wrote, "they make a perfect meal." Sometimes he ground the banana chips into a powder that could be transformed into biscuits. His banana biscuits blended "two parts banana flour and one part wheat flour." Gandhi preferred eating the uncooked banana powder along with dried mangoes. These provided him with an inexpensive, simple, and "most nourishing diet." Some raw enthusiasts would not see Gandhi's "uncooked" banana powder as raw, given his use of the sun in its preparation. While he strove to increase the percentage of foods he ate uncooked, he rarely approached raw food with the obsessive anxiety he brought to his struggles with sweets and dairy.[6]

Gandhi was not alone in his experiments with raw food. Uncooked vegetables were a staple for many of his vegetarian friends. When T. R. Allinson reassured him that he did not need milk to recover from his illness in London, raw vegetables were a key part of the alternative remedy. "The vegetables were not to be cooked but merely grated fine," Gandhi explained, "if I could not masticate them." He tried the raw diet for three days before returning to cooked food. "My body was not in a condition to enable me to do full justice to the experiment," he stated. Like Gandhi, Allinson believed in the power of raw food without being a zealot. He published a lengthy vegetarian cookbook, complete with recipes that called for heating. Perhaps Gandhi tried Allinson's recipe for almond pudding, baked apple custard, boiled asparagus, or herb pie. Before he embraced extreme simplicity in diet, he followed his vegetarian colleagues in sampling a great variety of delicacies.[7]

Many of his favorite treats did not require cooking. Millie Polak witnessed the mahatma hosting friends at the Westminster Palace Hotel in London. At the beginning of the culinary ritual, "newspapers would be spread over the table, and piles of oranges, apples, bananas, perhaps grapes, and a big bag of unshelled monkey- or pea-nuts, would be put ready." After tea arrived, the feast would begin. "Some would walk about or stand," Polak remembered, "and the nut-shells would fly around the room, orange juice would run over the paper-covered table, and at the end of the meal the room looked rather as if an ill-bred party of schoolboys had been let loose in it."[8]

Such revelry should not obscure the radical nature of Gandhi's turn away from cooking. Rejecting British rule, stripping away Western clothes, forsaking sex—all these were moderate compared to Gandhi's greatest renunciation. To give up cooking in the land of *palak paneer, dal makhani, idli sambar,* and *bhindi masala*—that was radical indeed. As a young man, Gandhi took pride in the marvels of Indian cooking. "It is needless to say," he declared, "that India would far outbid France in cooking vegetables nicely." Devotees of French cooking would disagree vehemently. Gandhi's point had less to do with French food than with his patriotic devotion to the culinary arts of his native land. That devotion helps to explain why he never totally abandoned cooking, just as he did not fully abandon flavor. The flavors of India, and especially of Gujarat, called for cooking—and those flavors were too close to his heart to be entirely forsaken.[9]

Gandhi's interest in raw food inspired him to cook less and to cook wisely. He recognized that the flavor of some foods could be harmed by cooking. "It is a waste of money and 'good' taste to cook these leaves or tubers," he wrote of radishes, turnips, and carrots. "The uncooked vegetables have a natural good taste of their own which is destroyed by cooking." Eating his vegetables raw was only the beginning. Over time, he hoped "to replace cooked items with uncooked articles and wheat by nuts."[10]

In June 1929, at the age of fifty-nine, Gandhi launched a public experiment with raw food. For over a month, he eliminated all cooked food from his diet and reported the results in his newspaper. He ate almonds, grated coconut, green leafy vegetables, raisins, lemons, and honey. He was especially excited by the possibilities of sprouted wheat and gram. He offered his readers instructions on how to sprout their own: "If wheat or gram is soaked in water for 24 hours and then the water is strained and it is then kept in a piece of wet cloth overnight, it sprouts." Before this experiment, Gandhi had cooked his cereals and pulses out of concern that they would be impossible to digest raw. Sprouts allowed him to gain the benefits of grains and beans without worrying about digestion.[11]

Gandhi's new experiment at first proved successful. Eating raw food did not impede his active life. "There has been no obstacle in my incessant activities," he declared. On the contrary, his diet helped him cope with stress. His systolic blood pressure had been consistently above 155. After beginning his raw diet, it dropped to 118. He also lost five pounds. High in fiber and low in calories, most raw diets lead to weight loss. For many of us, the loss of five pounds would be good news. For Gandhi, it was cause for concern. He was already bone thin, and returned reluctantly to eating cooked food.[12]

Eating raw food was similar to not drinking milk—a dietary ideal Gandhi never fully realized. Still, he believed his raw food experiments were "very important," not just for himself but for all of Indian society. By reducing the need for cooking fuel and cooking oil, a raw diet promised economic savings. "There is no need to eat food fried in ghee or oil," he wrote in 1942. Eating raw also involved less time in the kitchen. Rather than eating at a restaurant, Gandhi preferred to prepare his own meals, even if that entailed cooking. In 1918, he told his son, "It is true that cooking takes some time but I believe that this time is not wasted." Still, Gandhi believed in minimizing his time in the kitchen, explaining to his son that he often made soup, as he could sit and read while it cooked. In Yeravda jail in 1932, he took an active interest in the most efficient way to steam lentils. Going raw was even more of a time-saver. Advocates of "slow food" argue for a return to traditional methods of cooking and eating that prioritize flavor and quality over expediency. By contrast, Gandhi's desire to liberate India's poor led him to seek his own version of fast food. To the poor, a little extra money or an extra hour every day could open up a path to a better life. The liberating potential of a raw diet inspired Gandhi to opine that raw food had "a value not merely sanitary but also economic and moral or spiritual."[13]

Gandhi's raw utopia would emancipate not only India's poor but also its women. If cooking could be avoided, he suggested, "much of the time of our womenfolk . . . would then be saved." Once India had gone raw, he predicted, "women will be set free from the prison-house of the kitchen." Importantly, Gandhi did not equate cooking with oppression. If someone loved to cook, they should be free to do so. What he opposed was a system in which women were forced to cook. By reducing the time necessary to prepare meals, he hoped, a raw diet could liberate women and return the kitchen to its rightful status as a place of joyful creation.[14]

Gandhi was not alone in striving to free women from the tedium of traditional food preparation. The first half of the twentieth century witnessed many culinary reforms that promised to free women from cooking. Most of these efforts failed to envision a broader liberation from the constraints of patriarchy. Gandhi's views on women were complex. He often made decisions for his wife and, as we have seen, allowed only men to join the Salt March. At the same time, he argued that women should have leadership positions in the struggle to free India from British rule. As the feminist scholar Madhu Kishwar has written, "Gandhi saw women not as objects of reform and humanitarianism but as self-conscious subjects who could, if they choose, become arbiters of their own destiny."[15]

Just as Gandhi pursued multiple goals—the unity of India, the end of poverty, the liberation of women—he juggled multiple dietary changes in pursuit of those goals. He combined his "saltless," vegetarian, and raw food diets. Note the preponderance of raw foods in this description of his saltless menu: "papaw, 20 dates, four oranges, two sour limes, four dessert-spoonfuls honey, one lb. goat's milk, one dessert-spoonful almond paste." Raw, low-salt foods, all vegetarian, mostly fruits and nuts—this was the core of Gandhi's diet. His ultimate aim in pioneering a raw diet was the same goal that motivated him to give up salt while attacking the salt tax—freeing India from British rule, and the poverty and violence that defined that rule.[16]

Gandhi strove to use his diet to bring *swaraj* to every Indian. He failed. Poverty and injustice survived the end of British rule. There is good evidence that Gandhi helped to reduce poverty, and to strengthen Indian democracy. Yet many of his efforts, including his dietary experiments, proved dramatically less successful than he had hoped. He inspired some people to experiment with raw food—but despite his efforts, a raw food mass movement failed to materialize.[17]

Today, raw food is undergoing a renaissance. Restaurants specializing in raw food have sprouted in cities throughout America. Gandhi would likely have had mixed feelings about the recent surge of interest in eating raw. Raw food often attracts affluent foodies; in tragic contrast to Gandhi's vision, the poor are the least likely to eat large amounts of raw food, largely because poor neighborhoods lack access to fresh fruits and vegetables. Such food deserts are common in American cities. In India, the poor often struggle to gain access to sufficient food of any kind. Gandhi hoped that raw food would undo the inequalities that prevent poor people from having access to healthy food. Instead, those inequalities have prevented poor people from accessing raw food. Gandhi's raw utopia remains to be achieved.[18]

NATURAL VIRTUE

Gandhi's belief in the power of uncooked food did not blind him to the challenge of eating it. He advised patience when beginning a raw diet. "In the beginning stages," he noted, "there will probably be a feeling of emptiness." He explained such emptiness as a result of "the fact that by ill usage the stomach is distended." "Till it assumes its natural size," he advised, "the emptiness should be put up with." Those suffering from an empty belly could cope "by taking juicy fruit or a little more vegetable or better still by drinking plenty of water."[19]

Even for Gandhi, avoiding cooked foods was not easy. In 1914, in the midst of an experiment with raw food, he wrote a friend that "the temptation to take cooked fruit was great." With every dietary experiment, he learned new ways to cope with temptation. He also learned that patience was necessary to any lasting dietary change. To improve his patience, as well as his digestion, he turned to one of the most undervalued aspects of eating—chewing.[20]

"It is out of our ignorance that we believe we get our bread because of our efforts," Gandhi wrote from the deck of a British ship in 1909. "He who has given us teeth will also give us food for chewing." Gandhi believed in chewing. "Too much stress cannot be laid on the great necessity of thorough mastication," he declared. To a prominent Indian public figure, he wrote, "Every morsel of diet must be chewed with deliberation so that it goes down the throat not as a solid mass but as a smooth thick liquid." The nineteenth century produced many prophets of mastication; perhaps the most famous, Horace Fletcher, defended thorough chewing so ardently that his name became associated with the practice. Advocates of "fletcherizing" claimed that the act increased nutrient absorption and decreased indigestion. Fletcher himself assumed the title "the great masticator."[21]

Gandhi praised raw foods for inspiring "better mastication," and encouraged the eating of bread without sauces or curries in order to maximize chewing. Chomping his dry chapati, Gandhi risked turning the joy of eating into a mechanical process of digestion, but he did not see it that way. For him, chewing was more than an effective aid to digestion; it was also an apt metaphor for his deliberative approach to diet.[22]

Gandhi's belief in raw foods and in chewing coincided with a strong distrust of industrial processing. Prepared in factories far from the consumer, processed foods diminish the connection between the ingredients of a meal and the person eating that meal. They are, in effect, pre-chewed. "Almost all processed foods are adulterated," Gandhi wrote in 1909. In language that applies equally well today, he declared, "Big factories preparing items like jelly engage expert chemists who are expected to give to inferior products the appearance of quality goods." The pursuit of profit drove food processors to ignore the dangers of their products. "The producers," Gandhi wrote, "have their eyes only on profit and never care what harm they do to people." Categorically, he declared, "processed foods must never be used."[23]

Gandhi embraced simple whole foods: the fewer the ingredients, the better. Recently, markets have begun to fill with products that cater to such simple tastes. Ice cream brands boast less than five ingredients. Peanut butter revels in being solely peanuts and salt. This turn toward simplicity continues an ancient culinary fascination with purity. The food historian Sidney Mintz has examined the demand for pure food through the lens of marzipan, the sweet almond paste often used in desserts. Marzipan straddles the divide between processed and unprocessed, and thus reveals the complex and contradictory nature of purity itself. "By 'pure' we do mean natural, unspoiled, simple, earthy," Mintz explains, "but by 'pure' we also mean safe, biologically cleansed, scientifically aseptic, germ-free. The contrast in meaning centers on two rather dissimilar views of nature which, perhaps oddly, many of us appear to hold simultaneously."[24]

Gandhi defended the pure and the natural, even while new technologies reshaped how consumers understood those keywords. He lived through the rise of processed food, and his life highlights an overlooked dimension of the history of food processing—the role of empire. Food scholar Jayeeta Sharma has mapped the growth of "new agro-industrial foods across networks of imperial knowledge and commodity circulation." Worcestershire sauce, for example, was developed in India but became a staple throughout the British Empire. The link between packaged commodities and imperialism went well beyond processed food. Within the imperial machine, India itself became a product to be packaged and consumed. Just as processing eliminates natural variety, so imperial foodways condensed the many foods of India into an overly simplified caricature of the exotic. In 1747, Hannah Glasse offered the first English recipe to make "a currey in the indian way." The word "curry," from the Tamil for "sauce," began as a generic reference to many different kinds of Indian dishes. Much was lost as *curry* took on its singular status as the marker of a generic Indian food stripped of its regional varieties.[25]

From the beginning, the food processing industry had imperial ambitions. Food was changed so that it could be more easily packaged, preserved, and shipped to the far corners of the globe. Gandhi's anticolonialism dovetailed with his opposition to processed food, much of which was imported from abroad. As a young man, Gandhi had been inspired by the *swadeshi* movement and its boycotts of foreign goods (*swadeshi* means "from one's own *desh* or country"). In opposition to imperial processed food, he launched his own culinary *swadeshi* movement. He targeted one of the first manufactured foods to be imported into India on a large scale—margarine.

Long before butter substitutes became a popular staple in the Western world, Gandhi railed against their arrival in India, where they were often called "vegetable ghee." His opposition to vegetable ghee is especially remarkable given his profound desire to find vegan alternatives to anything made from cow's milk. "Though I yield to none in my enthusiasm for vegetarianism," Gandhi wrote, "I could never bring myself to use the chemically doctored vegetable product which is generally palmed off on the gullible public as ghee." The way in which such margarine was "chemically treated" made it "injurious to health" and "worthless as a food." It was not processing per se, but industrial or chemical processing that Gandhi opposed. Indeed, he encouraged his readers to produce their own chemical-free margarine. "Everyone in India," he wrote, "can prepare for himself good vegetable ghee from an undried cocoanut which can be procured cheap in any bazaar." The earliest forms of margarine, stuffed with dangerous trans fats, have proven to be more unhealthy than the butter they were meant to replace. Gandhi did not know about trans fats. His opposition to margarine stemmed from his belief that industrial processing yielded unhealthy food.[26]

As foods became loaded with additives and preservatives, Gandhi steered his diet in the opposite direction—toward unprocessed foods with as few ingredients as possible. He had always prized simplicity. In 1905, he chastised a relative for sending sweets. "I am anxious," he explained, "not to introduce complex dishes in the house." He was not completely opposed to culinary complexity. In the same letter, he mentioned sending "two loaves of Kuhne, biscuits, sweets, cake and *papad*," a traditional Indian dish that he described as follows: "dry, crisp and paperlike, it is made from a variety of pulses and spices." Sweets and *papad* do not indicate an especially strict austerity, but Gandhi's reference to Kuhne bread reveals the direction of his dietary preferences. Inspired by Louis Kuhne, the German naturopath, Kuhne bread was made from unleavened whole grains. In 1906, Gandhi praised a colleague for "living a very simple life" and eating food that "is likewise simple." "For example," he wrote, "last evening he only had bread, butter, *papad* and cocoa for dinner, and walked with me three-and-a-half miles before turning in for the night." Over time, Gandhi's definition of the "simple life" would grow more stark. "Formerly, people had two or three meals consisting of homemade bread and vegetables," he wrote in *Hind Swaraj*. "Now, they require something to eat every two hours so that they have hardly leisure for anything else." Gandhi's critique of excessive consumption inspired him to restrict his own diet in ever more creative ways.[27]

In 1915, he recorded the following in his diary: "Vow to have in India only five articles of food during 24 hours, and that before sunset. Water not included in five articles. Cardamom, etc., included. Groundnut and its oil to count as one article." Limiting his daily diet to five items proved salutary. "My health is excellent," he wrote a few years later. "My food is milk and oranges and one green vegetable plain boiled without salt." When available, he also savored grapes and pomegranate seeds. But he stuck to only five foods per day. "My life is simpler than ever," he declared. Gandhi savored "living on goat's milk and bread and raisins," and did not regret his "vow not to take more than five things." His use of a vow signals the spiritual dimension of his turn toward simple food. Counting and restricting the number of foods consumed is yet another form of Jain asceticism. While Gandhi's commitment to eating only five foods per day waxed and waned over the course of his life, such simplicity remained the lodestar of his spiritual approach to diet. In his words, "Experience suggests that as we start leading a simple life and as we become firm in our search for self-realisation, our craving for variety in food dwindles."[28]

Gandhi's austere simplicity might not appeal to today's champions of "real" food. Consumers are turning toward organic products with fewer ingredients, but they still demand variety and flavor. Few would be happy eating only five things per day. Even Gandhi struggled with such a restriction. He admitted, "The mind, the dog that it still is, runs about like one seeking to extract the utmost relish from the five articles."[29]

Limiting his diet inspired Gandhi to pay careful attention to everything he ate. Such attention helped him avoid preservatives and additives. It is not easy to decide when processed food is harmful; indeed, it is difficult to even define "processed" food. Many traditional foods—from yogurt and cheese to bread and oatmeal—require some sort of processing. When Gandhi cautioned against eating "ready-made" foods, he used jaggery, a kind of sugar, as an example. To make jaggery, he explained, "sugar-cane juice is boiled and from the whole only the sugar or jaggery is retained." He opposed such processing, and not just for sugar. "If mangoes were to be processed in the same manner," he declared, "the product would likewise be unacceptable." Jaggery has been embraced by many health-conscious consumers as a relatively unprocessed form of sugar. Unlike standard table sugar, jaggery retains the nutrient-rich molasses and has been neither bleached nor homogenized. What is processed for one person is "natural" or even "raw" for another.[30]

Consider the debate over pasteurization. Named after Louis Pasteur, the process prevents bacterial infection by bringing milk to a high temperature and then quickly cooling and sealing it. Gandhi decried the dangers of infected milk, but his belief in raw food inspired him to experiment with unboiled milk. "I began yesterday to take unboiled fresh milk," he reported in 1933. "They say," he explained, "that unboiled milk if fresh and clean is any day preferable to and more digestible than boiled milk." From jail, he wrote a colleague to suggest a diet of raw vegetables and "two and a half ounces of unboiled milk." Today, many health-conscious consumers have returned, like Gandhi, to raw milk; they believe it contains nutrients that are destroyed by the pasteurization process, and are willing to assume the risk of contamination.[31]

Gandhi was not opposed to all ways of processing food. He encouraged traditional methods that made the most of abundant staples like the coconut. Throughout much of India, coconut meat was often dried in order to make copra, a hardy substance that could be kept for long periods before being pressed for its oil. After instructing one correspondent to "make copra or ground-nut oil at home," Gandhi clarified that this should be done using "the indigenous grinding stones." He also suggested "crushing fresh cocoanut kernel to a fine paste and straining it through a piece of cloth" in order to produce coconut milk and coconut ghee.[32]

From milk to peanut butter to coconut ghee, deciding how much to process his food forced Gandhi to grapple with his values. One guiding principle emerged: home processing was categorically different from industrial processing. Crushing and straining your own coconuts was superior to buying a can of coconut milk. How much should food be processed, even at home? That question was more difficult for Gandhi to answer, especially when it came to the only staple of his diet that he struggled to eat raw: whole grains.

THE TRUE STAFF OF LIFE

After fruits, vegetables, and nuts, Gandhi's favorite food group was grains. Unlike fruits, grains require at least some degree of "processing." You cannot easily eat raw wheat. In 1914, Gandhi wrote his son that he had failed to live "on just dry fruits." He would have to "keep wheat" in his diet. The wheat kernel or berry contains three parts—the rough bran, the rich germ, and the calorie-packed endosperm. White bread consists of endosperm alone. Gandhi rejected such an impoverished form of wheat. In order to retain the nutrition of the bran and the wheat germ, he soaked whole wheat berries in water for twelve hours and then roasted them. "I thought they would pop up," he wrote. Instead, they "became hard." Never one to end an experiment early, Gandhi added hot milk and sugar (his opposition to sweeteners not withstanding) and continued to cook the mixture until it "became gruel." "Chewing it took a lot of time," he reported. Happily, the necessity of chewing never harmed Gandhi's enjoyment of a meal. He ate his wheat gruel "with relish."[33]

Over time, Gandhi refined his recipe for wheat porridge. The basics remained the same: whole wheat berries soaked overnight and then roasted. The roasted berries were then coarsely ground and boiled to a "silken fine" paste. Gandhi suggested adding "a little ghee" to the paste while it boiled and then serving it with milk. The goal, in his words, was "a thick *khichdi*-like paste." A Gujarati staple made with rice and lentils, *khichdi* resembles Gandhi's wheat porridge in its hearty healthfulness as well as its mushy texture. It was, for Gandhi, the ultimate comfort food. When Mahadev Desai, Gandhi's longtime personal secretary, expressed concern that he had done something wrong, Gandhi reassured him, "It is for your efficiency and your character that I have chosen you to help me in my political work and you have not disappointed me. Add to this the fact that you can cook *khichdi* for me, with so much love." *Khichdi* embodies the Gujarati roots of Gandhi's emotional connection to food. That he would choose it to describe the consistency of his porridge reveals his desire to link his experiments back to the culinary world of his youth and of his compatriots. He wanted as wide an audience as possible for his wheat porridge. Writing in 1912, before he abandoned sweets, he suggested dressing up the dish "with honey or some home-made jam."[34]

Many of Gandhi's vegetarian friends embraced porridge as the culinary embodiment of simple rural values. Long seen as the coarse fodder of commoners, the staple made a dramatic return throughout Europe in the last decades of the nineteenth century. As the romantic poets celebrated uncivilized nature, food reformers exalted the traditional, the rustic, and the authentically rural. Porridge fit perfectly. To improve his recipe, Gandhi bought a coffee mill and began to grind roasted wheat berries into a powder. He soaked the powder in water and milk for ten minutes and then added "a pinch of salt and a spoon of butter." Grinding the wheat rendered a finer, more easily consumed dish and also avoided the necessity of soaking the wheat berries. Like many modern chefs, Gandhi strove to save time while preparing delicious, nutritious meals. With ground whole wheat powder as one component, he declared, "one can very easily prepare the best food in ten minutes."[35]

Gandhi's passion for porridge did not prevent him from enjoying wheat in its most hallowed form—bread. Not just any bread would do, however. Gandhi joined an international movement to revive the art of baking whole grain loaves. Beginning in the early nineteenth century, forward-thinking dietary reformers had worried about the declining quality of bread. In the United States, Reverend Sylvester Graham denounced the common practice of removing the fibrous bran and treating the remaining flour with various chemicals. He developed his own whole meal bread, and complained that most people ate "the most miserable trash that can be imagined, in the form of bread, and never seem to think that they can possibly have anything better." Graham's name continues to adorn his most lasting invention: the graham cracker, designed as a healthy wholegrain snack, and later reengineered to suit the mass market. Graham would be aghast to learn that his cracker now consists mostly of white flour and sugar.[36]

In the early 1870s, a few years after Gandhi was born, a new revolution roiled the world of baking. For centuries, grains like wheat had been ground between stones. The heavy stones crushed wheat berries, separating out the fibrous bran but not the nutrient-rich germ. Mashed in with the energy-dense endosperm, the germ stained the flour with yellow carotenoids. The resulting flour suffered more than a peculiar color. The oil in the germ, susceptible to spoiling, dramatically shortened the shelf life of the flour. Searching for a way to purify and preserve wheat flour, bakers turned to smooth rollers made of porcelain, iron, or steel. Able to separate the germ as well as the bran, the new rollers left behind only the white, long-lasting endosperm. Thus, white bread was born. Seemingly more pure and undoubtedly longer lasting, white flour quickly won admirers. But replacing coarse ground flour with white flour led to outbreaks of mysterious illnesses, later identified as pellagra and beri-beri, both caused by vitamin deficiencies. The same wheat germ that tinted flour and caused it to spoil quicker also contained an array of vital nutrients. Bakers could have healthy bread or white bread, but they could not have both.[37]

For much of Gandhi's life, the nutritional deficiencies of white bread were not widely acknowledged. Nutritional experts arrayed themselves on both sides of what became a contentious debate over the ideal flour. Most of Gandhi's friends joined forces against white bread. His vegetarian doctor, T. R. Allinson, gained fame as an advocate of whole grain baking. His manifesto, *The Advantages of Wholemeal Bread*, published in 1889, claimed not only that whole meal was superior to white but that it was the ideal food, "the true staff of life." Gandhi became an avid fan of Allinson's whole meal and of the idea that whole grains were especially nutritious. Traveling by ship a few months after the beginning of the First World War, he taught the ship's baker how to make whole grain bread. "I asked him to whip the water before adding it to the flour," he wrote a friend. "This aerates the bread and makes it very light." He added that it was "Allinson's meal" that he used on board the ship.[38]

Allinson galvanized an international movement to save bread from the evils of overly processed flour. Like Sylvester Graham, he blended his love for whole wheat with other social and political reforms. Role models for Gandhi, both Graham and Allinson believed that reforming what people ate would revolutionize how they lived. They were not alone. No one had more ambitious hopes for the whole grain movement than the dynamic secretary of the Bread Reform League, May Yates. Yates reinforced Gandhi's love for whole grains while providing him with a model of dietary activism. A respected painter who exhibited her work in the Royal Academy, she was an equally talented organizer and a fiery speaker. She sold her jewels to launch the Bread Reform League and championed her causes across Europe and the United States. In addition to whole grains, she promoted vegetarianism and attacked alcohol. Her Bread Reform League later merged with the London Vegetarian Society, strengthening the connections between two of Gandhi's culinary pillars. Yates used India to demonstrate the superiority of a vegetarian, whole grain diet. "Experience shows that those nations who do not eat meat," she wrote, "almost invariably adopt brown bread." For an example, she turned to "the Hindoos of the North-Western Provinces" who "can walk fifty or sixty miles a day with no other food than 'chapaties' made of whole-meal with a little 'ghee' or Galam butter."[39]

Inspired by Allinson and Yates, Gandhi joined the whole grain movement. In one of his first articles on diet, published in 1891, he praised the "poor classes" in India for eating the "coarsest bran." Such coarse flour was, he argued, "far superior to the ordinary flour that is used here for the much-abused white bread." Gandhi dismissed white flour as "innutritious," "injurious," and "insipid." In South Africa, he encouraged his followers to grind their wheat at home. If they did not feel like bread, they could make porridge. "If well cooked in water and taken with milk or sugar," he stated, wheat porridge "tastes delicious and is much superior to other kinds of food." Decades later, in 1942, he repeated his belief that cereals and grains should be ground at home and eaten whole. Sieving the flour risked removing "a rich source of salts and vitamins."[40]

Although he remained critical of white flour throughout his life, Gandhi distanced himself from the more extreme advocates of whole grains. "One army of doctors defended white bread for all they were worth," he later recalled, "and another army suggested that white bread was the staff of death and that the brown bread alone was the staff of life." Both sides were "fanatical" and made "absolute conclusions" without "sufficient data." Whole wheat was preferable to white flour, but it was not a panacea.[41]

While bakers fought over whether to use white or whole wheat flour, another nutritional debate centered on whether to use wheat at all. In recent times, the protein in wheat known as gluten has earned a bad reputation. In the 1950s, gluten was linked to celiac disease, a condition that requires completely avoiding the protein. Now, many people claim degrees of sensitivity to gluten that range from mild to severe. Increasingly, gluten-free labels have become commonplace. In Gandhi's day, by contrast, gluten was renowned not only for the elasticity it gave bread but also for its nutritional benefits. Indeed, wheat protein played a key role in an imperialist narrative that divided the people of India into "hearty" wheat-eating northerners and "weak" rice-eating southerners.

Colonel Robert McCarrison, Gandhi's old antagonist concerning the merits of vegetarian food, gave a scientific veneer to the colonial preference for wheat. He fed different groups of rats what he understood to be the diets of different regions of India, and found "a marked decline in their vitality as the northern diet of wheat and meat gave way to one based on rice and vegetables." He used this disparity to explain the difference between "the manly, stalwart and resolute races of the north" and "the poorly developed, toneless and supine people of the east and south." Field Marshal Colin Campbell, commander in chief of the Indian Army, and Major David McCay, professor at Calcutta Medical College, concurred that wheat was key to the health of the so-called martial races. This was the same McCay who linked the absence of protein to "a cringing effeminate disposition." Yet again, he wielded racial stereotypes to buttress his nutritional dogma. According to McCay, a diet based on rice left Bengalis with "slackness, want of vigour, tonelessness," as well as "little power of attention, observation, or concentration of thought." The British preference for wheat even worked its way into a Rudyard Kipling story. Entitled "William the Conqueror," the story follows a colonial official striving to end famine in South India. When the locals, accustomed to rice, refuse to eat wheat, the official gives the hearty grain to goats and then uses their milk to feed starving babies. Thus, Kipling endorsed wheat and the humanitarian creativity of British officials while painting South Indians as ignorant and weak.[42]

Gandhi inherited the British preference for wheat over rice. His criticism of rice—that most hallowed of Indian grains—avoided the racial imperialism of McCarrison and Kipling. Instead, Gandhi focused on nutrition. He noted that many doctors blamed rice for "the diabetes from which the Bengalees very often suffer." "No one in India would call rice a nourishing food," he declared. "It is the food of the rich, i.e., of people who do not want to work." Although he would always prefer wheat, Gandhi's opinion of rice softened with time. Like wheat, rice can be prepared in ways that preserve its nutritional content. Rice contains a hard outer layer that has to be removed. Gandhi encouraged pounding off this layer by hand so as not to damage the nutritious pericarp. "Machine-pounding," he explained, "not only removes the outer skin, but also polishes the rice by removing its pericarp." Unpolished brown rice was, Gandhi suggested, far healthier than the more popular varieties of white rice. When a friend complained that brown rice was filling, Gandhi responded with a lecture on the fundamentals of diet and nutrition. "Our object," he retorted, "is not to fill the belly with as much as can be put into it, but to take a proper proportion of balanced foods." Eating whole grains helps achieve such a healthy balance; by contrast, white rice offers too many calories without sufficient protein and fiber. Without the nutritious pericarp, "polished rice is practically starch."[43]

Gandhi limited his starch intake. "Among fresh vegetables, a fair amount of leafy vegetables must be taken every day," he wrote. "I do not include potatoes, sweet potatoes, *suran* etc., which supply starch mainly." Gandhi overlooked the many nutritional benefits of the sweet potato. More akin to a carrot than a potato, the sweet potato contains an abundance of beta-carotene, vitamin C, and other nutrients. *Suran*, also known as elephant foot yam, similarly deserves to be distinguished from the potato; the massive tuber (hence the name) provides a range of vitamins. Gandhi knew that starchy vegetables often contained nutrients. Even his beloved banana contained a lot of starch. "Banana is a good fruit," he wrote. "But as it is very rich in starch," he added, "it takes the place of bread." He advised one correspondent, "You should take in liberal quantities of leafy vegetables and gourds. Of starchy vegetables you should take only a little or none at all."[44]

Gandhi praised whole grains for helping prevent constipation. "The pericarp also supplies roughage," he explained, "which helps the action of the bowels." For those suffering from irregularity, he also provided a list of especially potent fruits: "figs, French plums, muscatel raisins, large grapes, black grapes, green grapes and oranges." Gandhi held up good digestion as a marker of a healthy diet and a healthy life. Consider his advice to pregnant women. "Her diet should be regular, easy to digest and nourishing," he wrote. "If she gets constipated," she should "increase the quantity of olive oil." If she suffered from nausea, on the other hand, "she should take lime juice in a little water without sugar." Gandhi's concern for the health of pregnant women inspired him to offer some marital advice. The ideal husband would not "agitate the wife by starting quarrels with her during this period." If the pregnant woman "has to carry too heavy a burden of domestic work, the husband should try to lighten it."[45]

As his advice to expecting couples makes clear, Gandhi often blended dietary advice with larger life lessons. Eating well was, after all, a means to living well. Once again, he made clear that a raw diet did not preclude the necessity of moderation and control of the palate. "A ripe fruit which has fallen off the tree, if eaten to gratify one's palate," he declared, "will be tainted food." By contrast, "a cooked meal of vegetables and cereals, prepared and served in the normal course, will be pure food if eaten to satisfy one's hunger and without any thought of gratifying the palate." Did healthy eating require such an extreme rejection of flavor? Would a ripe mango really be tainted if eaten for pleasure? As he had with salt and sugar, Gandhi approached whole foods with a Victorian austerity that negated the benefits of flavor. But as his love affair with fruit makes evident, he was not always consistent in rejecting flavor, especially when it came to his favorite breakfast.[46]

"EAT FRUIT"

At 5:15 in the morning of November 3, 1932, Gandhi was inspired to write a letter about his breakfast, a simple fruit salad that consisted of two sweet limes, two oranges, and the juice of a pomegranate. Gandhi added "a pinch of salt" to the pomegranate juice and poured the result over the limes and the oranges. "Writing of the fruit salad, I give you my discovery," he scribbled excitedly. "I find that fruit to produce the greatest effect should be taken by itself and on an empty stomach. You might almost say, the same law applies to juicy fruit that applies to opening medicines." Noting that the Sanskrit for food and medicine is the same word, *aushadh*, he stated, "all food should be taken as medicine"—carefully and in pursuit of health rather than flavor. In this instance, the healthiest of foods also happened to be the most delicious.[47]

Many of Gandhi's dietary principles could be boiled down to the advice he offered a wealthy industrialist in 1924: "Eat fruit." Throughout his life, fruit was at the heart of Gandhi's diet. "I take goat's milk twice and fruits thrice," he wrote in 1919. More than once, he experimented with what he understood as a pure fruit diet. His list of preferred fruits included not only bananas, oranges, dates, figs, apples, and pineapples, but also "almonds, walnuts, peanuts and coconuts." Such an inclusive definition of fruit helps to explain how Gandhi could conclude that fruits contain "all the elements necessary for health and energy." His belief in raw food fueled his passion for fruits and vegetables. He stressed that "scientists say that this food need not be cooked, and as animals maintain health by eating sun-ripened fruit, so should we."[48]

The nutritional benefits of fruit were paramount for Gandhi. "Chemists have shown by experiment," he wrote, "that fruits contain all the elements necessary for the maintenance of human life." The validity of that statement depended on the way he defined fruit, as well as the remarkable variety of fruits, vegetables, and nuts he consumed. Take, for example, this diet he suggested in 1915: "bananas, mangoes, oranges, oats, figs (fresh or dried), sultanas, grapes, lemons, tamarind, papaw, pineapple, prunes, cocoanut, groundnuts, almonds, pistachios, walnuts, olive oil, if necessary." Gandhi relished the diversity of fruits available in India. He recommended "mangoes, *jambu*, guavas, grapes, papaws, limes—sweet or sour—oranges, *mosambi*, etc." *Jambu*, a relative of guava, and *mosambi*, a kind of sweet lime, were included on the list even though he had also included guava and sweet lime. No fruit should go unrecognized.[49]

For six months in the winter of 1912 and 1913, Gandhi ate nothing but fruits and nuts. His diet consisted of "bananas, peanuts, olive oil, lemon or similar citrus fruit, and dates." Gandhi credited the diet with boosting his immune system. He also reported having increased "physical and mental energy." The experiment had not been totally successful; Gandhi could not lift as much weight as before. He could, however, "work for longer periods at a stretch without fatigue." He recommended the diet to others as "little short of miraculous."[50]

For the next few years, Gandhi spent many of his days "living on purely uncooked fruitarian food." He declared, "We are getting more convinced by experience every day that a fruit diet is the best." He perfected such delicacies as "banana flour and almond coffee," "banana flour and coconut biscuits," and "ground monkeynuts or dried bananas stewed." The stew he described as "a concession to Mrs. Gandhi and a temporary indulgence for my palate." Even Mrs. Gandhi "remained a pure fruitarian." "It is a most wonderful thing indeed," Gandhi concluded of his "pure fruit" diet.[51]

The wonders of this diet did not always include frugality. Gandhi lamented the cost of many fruits and vegetables. "If grape is dear," he told his son, "you can have raisins instead." In March 1913, he told a friend that he was eliminating one of the central pillars of his diet because it had become too expensive. "Cannot afford almonds," he wrote, "and do not want to eat them myself when I cannot share them with the children." Fresh fruit and nuts were not always expensive, however. After describing a diet that consisted primarily of "fresh fruit, wheat and olive oil," Gandhi noted, "Such a diet costs very little trouble or money."[52]

During a trip to Rangoon, Gandhi penned a detailed description of his "fruitarian" diet. He was traveling with his wife and a friend, Dr. Mehta. "At 10 a.m.," he wrote, "we take the first meal":

Mine and Mrs. Gandhi's consists of uncooked fruits and nuts.
Ground-nuts are roasted. My menu today was 4 bananas, 2 tiny
tomatoes, 1 tiny unripe mango chopped, 2 spoonfuls of grated fresh
coconut, 4 walnuts, perhaps 2 ounces of date, groundnut meal mixed,
1 naarangi, 2 slices of wretched melon, 2 lemons and a drink of
coconut water. Much the same will be taken at 5 p.m. Dr. Mehta joins
me in the fruitarian meal. He adds milk and almonds to the above.
Both of us walk about the Town barefoot. Mrs. Gandhi cooks unripe
bananas when she can get them. I have now no desire for cooked
bananas. Hitherto, there has been no difficulty about procuring fruits
and nuts. Several young men in different parts of the country are
trying the fruitarian diet. I have asked them to let me have results.

Mrs. Gandhi cooked her bananas. Dr. Mehta added almonds and milk.
Gandhi noted these dietary idiosyncrasies without condemnation.
Despite his nutritional evangelism, he remained respectful of the dietary
needs of different people. He was a food missionary but not a zealot. His
tolerance grew from his awareness of his own dietary imperfections.
When it came to dietary matters, he admitted, "my thinking is ahead of
my action."[53]

Gandhi recognized that pure *ahimsa* was impossible; even eating
fruits and vegetables involved violence. Whereas "every grain of wheat
will yield a plant," he reasoned, the "part of the date fruit which we eat
will not grow if planted." Eating wheat was more violent than eating
dates. Considered from such a perspective, peanuts were unethical but
olives were potentially ethical because they contain "a separable seed"
that might be planted. What of his beloved almonds? Gandhi had briefly
given them up due to their cost. Would his conscience lead him to eliminate almonds from his diet forever? Faced with such a loss, Gandhi
revised his ethical scale. The key question, he argued, was not whether a
potential plant was being destroyed when a seed was eaten, but whether
the existing plant was harmed in the process of harvesting the seed. "An
almond tree continues to flourish," he wrote, even after almonds are harvested. "The wheat plant," on the other hand, "once the grain has been
removed, is no better than a weed."[54]

Gandhi's rocky relationship with ginger reveals the depths, both literal and figurative, of his concern for all living beings. He loved ginger,

but he was concerned about the ethics of eating the potent roots. "The consumption of roots," he explained, "is thoroughly objectionable according to Jain principles." Jain tradition proscribes eating *anant'kāys*, or "infinite bodies," plants whose edible parts have the potential to create new plants. According to one Jain teacher, "When a man eats a root crop, he destroys infinite souls." Respectful of Jain principles and aware that eating a root could compromise a plant's survival, Gandhi nevertheless decided to try ginger. He loved its sharp spice, and decided to add a little ginger to the juice of the neem tree, a plant famous for its antibacterial qualities. Gandhi often brushed his teeth with a neem twig, a practice common in India. By combining ginger and neem, he created a concoction with a host of health benefits. Ginger's anti-inflammatory qualities make it especially appealing for anyone with allergies or arthritis. Gandhi focused, however, on the taste. After Mrs. Gandhi collected "some tender shoots of ginger," Gandhi "ate them for a day or two and relished them very much indeed." A few days later, however, he was "filled with compassion" for the ginger. Rather than thinking only of its taste or nutritional qualities, he came to see it as a vital piece of an independent being. He saw "souls in these pieces of ginger." "Deeply pained," he vowed to treat ginger "as forbidden" and to "avoid eating it as far as possible."[55]

Gandhi's sympathy for the lost souls of those ginger shoots inspired him to meditate on the limitations of even the most ethical diet. After pondering the ethics of eating seeds and roots, he concluded, "It is not possible to go very deep into this kind of argument." The purpose of such a debate was not to reach a place of ethical absolutism, but to recognize that some violence was inherent in all life, and to live as humbly and nonviolently as possible. "The basic principle," he argued, was that "one should make do with the fewest possible articles and in the smallest possible quantity." Gandhi remained self-critical as he warned against fetishizing any particular dietary trend. "A man who cooks a meal of just an ounce of rough-ground wheat and is free in five minutes," he wrote, "is far superior to the one who wrings (as I do) the utmost pleasure from a variety of fruits."[56]

Gandhi believed that the flavor of fruit distracted him from his higher calling, and yet he also believed that fruit was a pillar of healthy eating. In the end, he decided that what mattered was the motive behind his diet. Feasting on raw mangoes entailed greater waste—greater violence—than cooking a simple meal. Even as he perfected his raw fruitarian diet, he stayed focused on the principle that food should fuel service.

The social potential of a raw diet led Gandhi to explore the cheapest source of sustenance for the poor: wild food. Foraging for wild fruits and vegetables offered a low-cost source of nutrition. But the ethical complications he encountered with ginger remained, and not just in regard to the potential harm caused to wild plants by overharvesting. The greatest ethical challenge stemmed from the limitations of wild food as a remedy for poverty. If the goal was to end hunger, changes in diet would be insufficient if they were not linked to changes in land ownership and the distribution of wealth—changes that seemed as impossible as eating ginger nonviolently.

WILD WONDERS

"Vegetable should be served daily," Gandhi wrote in 1932. "Mostly it should be leaves." Even though they worked in the fields, many villagers had little access to leafy greens. Gandhi strove "to find out the simplest and cheapest foods that would enable villagers to regain lost health." He hoped that "the addition of green leaves to their meals will enable villagers to avoid many diseases from which they are now suffering." How could vegetables be produced in greater abundance and with less cost so that everyone could eat an abundance of healthy greens?[57]

In the winter of 1934–35, a resident of Gandhi's ashram brought him "a leaf that was growing wild among the Ashram grasses." "It was *luni*," Gandhi wrote. "I tried it, and it agreed with me." The underappreciated leafy green, known in English as purslane, tastes like an earthy arugula or a spicy spinach. When cooked, it adds flavor and nutrition to stir-fries, soups, or lentils. In addition to offering vitamins A, B, and C, as well as some protein, *luni* packs more omega-3 fatty acids than almost any other vegetable source. Its combination of nutrition and availability made it the ideal leafy green for the rural poor. Gandhi recommended it frequently and, in the process, embraced the larger principle that nutritious food need not always be grown. It could be found.[58]

Not long after he brought Gandhi that *luni* leaf, the knowledgeable ashram resident unveiled another wild vegetable known as *chakwat*.

Commonly known as white goosefoot, *chakwat* offers a variety of options to the chef. Its leaves can be eaten raw or cooked like spinach. The seeds of the plant are also nutritious, offering large amounts of protein like their better-known relative, quinoa. Unlike most grains, quinoa has substantial amounts of all essential amino acids, as well as healthy doses of magnesium and calcium. Long prized in South America, quinoa has become popular worldwide for its rich nutritional profile, high amounts of protein, and diverse culinary uses. The popularity of quinoa provides a cautionary note about the dark side of the global market for health foods. Demand in wealthy countries has driven up the price of quinoa beyond the point where many Andeans can afford the vital crop. Gandhi hoped that raw food would provide the poor a dietary safety net beyond the whims of the market; the soaring cost of quinoa demonstrates the need for such wild sources of sustenance.[59]

Gandhi's positive experiences with *luni* and goosefoot left him hungry for more wild greens. One by one, he sampled "the leaves of *sarsav*, *suva*, turnip-tops, carrot-tops, radish-tops and pea-plant leaves." *Sarsav*, or mustard, is a plant with a rich nutritional profile. Like broccoli and other cruciferous vegetables, mustard greens contain glucosinolates, natural sulfur-containing phytochemicals that have been studied for their ability to reduce cholesterol and prevent cancer. In addition, mustard greens contain substantial amounts of vitamin K, vitamin A, vitamin C, folate, manganese, and calcium. After mustard greens, Gandhi listed *suva*, or dill. The word *dill* comes from the Norse term for "to lull." Dill has long been associated with calming the stomach and the mind. In addition to calcium, iron, and magnesium, it is rich in flavonoids, the family of compounds that give plants their colors. Flavonoids used to be known as vitamin P; some evidence suggests they can help fight cancer.[60]

Gandhi did not know many of the health benefits of the wild plants he was trying, but he realized that wild food offered a way to diversify the diets of the rural poor. He recognized, in his words, "the nourishing properties of the innumerable leaves that are to be found hidden among the grasses that grow wild in India." Unlike mustard greens and dill, *luni* and goosefoot are often treated as weeds. Gandhi appreciated them even more due to their ability to grow without cultivation. Recognizing the culinary value of weeds, like choosing raw food, allowed him to criticize the modern tendency to overprepare, overprocess, and overproduce. Not unlike the words *organic, raw, whole,* or *fresh,* the meaning of *wild* has shifted over time and in relation to major changes in the production and distribution of food. Eating raw and gathering wild, Gandhi embodied the principles of the so-called paleo diet. Advocates of paleo eating champion what they believe our Paleolithic ancestors ate before the onset of agriculture—mostly meat, fish, and wild fruits and vegetables. Unlike most paleo advocates, Gandhi did not eat meat. Like many paleo proponents, though, he linked the ill effects of modern food to a larger critique of the modernization and mechanization of agriculture and of society more generally.[61]

Criticizing what others took to be progress, Gandhi connected his dietary reform to a broader rejection of many facets of the modern world—including modern medicine. In *Hind Swaraj,* he attacked Western doctors. By treating symptoms resulting from what Gandhi considered bad behavior, doctors allowed their patients to ignore the root causes of illness. Tellingly, Gandhi framed his critique of modern medicine in terms of food: "I overeat, I have indigestion, I go to a doctor, he gives me medicine. I am cured. I overeat again, I take his pills again. Had I not taken the pills in the first instance, I would have suffered the punishment deserved by me and I would not have overeaten again."[62]

In a society saturated with pharmaceutical drugs, in which the medical establishment continues to focus more on treatment than prevention, Gandhi's approach to healing has much to offer. He believed that proper nutrition could eliminate the majority of human ailments, and that many diseases could be treated with herbal remedies. Unlike the most extreme advocates of natural medicine, he strove to find a middle ground between traditional dietary approaches to health and the more scientifically rigorous practices of Western medicine. He learned from peasants in rural India and the latest scientific discoveries, all while remaining convinced that a wise diet was the foundation of a true and lasting health.

CHAPTER 5

Natural Medicine

Like a lost jewel that takes greater effort to find than it does to keep
it in the first instance, good health, once it is lost, costs much time
and effort to regain.

GANDHI, 1913

ON JANUARY 30, 1948, GANDHI WAS SHOT AND KILLED AS HE
walked towards his evening prayers. His assassin had close ties to
a network of religious extremists who believed in a fascist conception of
a Hindu India, a conception that Gandhi rejected as neither Hindu nor
Indian. The mahatma learned from a variety of people and traditions
while holding firm to his own values. In his words, "I do not want my
house to be walled in on all sides and my windows to be stuffed. I want
the cultures of all the lands to be blown about my house as freely as possible. But I refuse to be blown off my feet by any." Gandhi balanced openness with rootedness, curiosity with integrity. Nowhere are the fruits of
that balance more evident than in his approach to the relationship
between food, health, and medicine.[1]

At a prayer meeting in New Delhi, one month before he was assassinated, Gandhi paid tribute to a Muslim doctor, Hakim Ajmal Khan. By
praising Dr. Khan, Gandhi connected religious harmony to the unity of
different medical traditions. The renowned leader of a hospital and medical college in Delhi, Khan had blended ayurveda and unani, two ancient
forms of medical science, one associated with Hindus and the other with

Muslims. While religious violence swept across India, Gandhi found hope in Khan's medical pluralism and in the connections between ayurveda, unani, and other forms of medicine: homeopathy, naturopathy, and what we might call mainstream, Western, or allopathic medicine. All of these labels are problematic. Indeed, Gandhi's diet bridged the divide between "alternative" and "mainstream" medicine.[2]

For Gandhi, the most powerful connection between food and health did not involve treating illness but preventing it. For millennia, Indian doctors had used food to prevent illness. The ancient sage Charaka, often considered the founder of ayurveda, recognized the healing power of diet. "The life of all living beings is food," he wrote. "Complexity, clarity, good voice, long life, understanding, happiness, satisfaction, growth, strength and intelligence are all established in food." The modern medical establishment has also recognized the importance of diet. When it comes to prevention, in particular, many doctors would agree with Gandhi that a healthy diet can be the best medicine.[3]

Gandhi experimented with multiple healing traditions and dozens of remedies for everything from constipation to fever to chronic fatigue. Many of these remedies have attracted interest from doctors, and are being studied for their healing potential. Gandhi would be happy. He believed that rigorous scientific experiments are necessary to distinguish between natural remedies that work and those that are, in his words, "nothing short of humbug." His belief in science makes his pluralist approach to natural medicine especially worthy of emulation. While he strove to learn from all medical traditions, he continually praised what we might call "evidence-based medicine." He advocated a scientific natural medicine rooted in diet and in admitting and learning from mistakes.[4]

At his most austere, Gandhi proclaimed that food should be medicine, consumed without pleasure solely for the purpose of feeding the body. Medicalizing his diet trapped him in egocentric nutritionism and limited the impact of his experiments. His life reveals the paradox that the healthiest diets call us away from a single-minded preoccupation with health. Gandhi's austerity limited his ability to follow one of his most cherished dietary principles—that food is at its most nutritious when we allow it to nourish more than just our bodies.[5]

In medicine, as in food, Gandhi prized simplicity. "If anybody has a headache," he wrote, "he should have a mud-pack on the head and drink lots of water." He believed that medical treatments should be as uncomplicated and inexpensive as possible. Otherwise, not everyone would be able to use them. In Gandhi's day, the science of nutrition had yet to become big business. Food companies did not invest in studies to prove the nutritional advantages of their wares. Edible "products" were only just beginning to be redesigned in order to manifest as many nutritional buzzwords as possible. Gandhi embraced the idea of nutrients, and his diet reveals the dangers of nutritionism. Sometimes, however, his natural approach to diet and health was as simple as a glass of water or a fistful of mud.[6]

Like many of his peers, Gandhi saw in the advance of nutritional science the possibility of a perfect diet—perfect, that is, from the perspective of health. Nothing inspired the dream of a nutritional utopia more than the discovery of vitamins, nutrients without which a human being cannot achieve full health. Today, many doctors argue that a balanced diet is sufficient to provide all the vitamins most people need. By contrast, advocates of multivitamins defend what they see as nutritional insurance. Gandhi died before the debate over vitamin supplements took its current form, but the larger issue of vitamin deficiency became a major concern during his lifetime and strongly influenced his thinking on many dietary questions. Importantly, his approach to vitamins focused not on supplements but on how to gain the maximum nutrition from food. Even more importantly, he highlighted the needs of the poor, those who are least likely to have access to vitamin supplements but are also most likely to need them.[7]

Although Gandhi became interested in nutrients as early as 1916, the word *vitamin* did not become central to his vocabulary until the middle of the 1920s. Even then, he used the word as a general term for "nutrients." In August 1926, he reported that milk provided "the finest vitamins." He noted that these vitamins were destroyed by boiling and were "considered essential for health," but he neither named the vitamins nor explained how they were essential. The next year, he wrote an American friend, Richard Gregg, about a mixture of goat's milk, neem leaf juice, and "hot raisin water." He explained that the mixture gave him "the vitamins from the milk" as well as "the vitamins from the neem leaves." He did not specify which vitamins came from the milk and which from the neem. To his credit, though, he made clear his desire to learn more. He sent Gregg a bevy of questions: "At what point are vitamins destroyed when you boil leafy vegetables? What is the virtue of vitamins? What is the quantity of leafy vegetables one should take in order to get the required measure of vitamins? What quantity of unboiled milk will give the vitamins required? Is it true that mere heating the milk does not destroy vitamins? Or they are only destroyed when milk is brought to the boiling point?" Gandhi's questions are revealing. He recognized his need for basic information, and dwelled on practical matters. He did not, however, ask how many vitamins existed, or what role different vitamins played in the body. Gandhi's lifetime of correspondence offers hundreds of references to vitamins, but many of those references lack specificity. He often used *vitamin* as a synonym for "nutrient."[8]

Gregg would play a key role in inspiring the use of Gandhian nonviolence in the American civil rights movement—but before he helped Dr. Martin Luther King Jr. learn about Gandhi, he helped Gandhi learn about vitamins. Gregg recommended a book, *Food, Health, Vitamins*, that had emerged two years earlier with the simpler title *Food and Health*. The change in title reveals the surge of interest in vitamins that had inspired Gandhi to contact Gregg in the first place. Gandhi read the work carefully. He deemed it "a good book" but rejected its emphasis on meat and its dismissal of legumes and nuts. In typical fashion, he used the absence of data to drive home his point: "The authors could not possibly have sufficient data about the effect of nuts and pulses to enable them to come to a just decision." Gandhi decided to seek his own evidence. Soon after receiving Gregg's letter, he asked an Indian doctor, M. S. Kelkar, if he had studied "the newest researches made about vitamins."[9]

As Gandhi learned more about vitamins, he began to share his knowledge. "We get from uncooked vegetables the nutrients that we require," he told readers of his Gujarati newspaper. "They are known as 'vitamins' in English, and doctors claim that these vitamins are destroyed as a result of cooking, and that their destruction leads to ill-health." Gandhi's burgeoning understanding reinforced his belief in raw food. He regularly stated that cooking destroyed vitamins. Although he continued to refer to vitamins in the abstract, he developed a particular interest in vitamin A. He also began to distinguish between nutrients in general and the vitamins that were especially essential for health. In 1929, he reported, "It is the opinion of contemporary Western medical men that our diet should contain a certain element in the absence of which a man cannot preserve his health. It is known as 'vitamin.' Vitamin means the vital essence. Chemists cannot detect it by analysis. But health experts have been able to feel its absence."[10]

Gandhi's belief in evidence led him to repeatedly revise his views. In 1929, he surmised that sunlight might provide "the most important of the vitamins." Gandhi's sunny hypothesis attracted the attention of his old interlocutor, Sir Robert McCarrison, whose belief in the supremacy of wheat over rice and of meat over vegetables does not accord with contemporary science. On vitamins, by contrast, McCarrison had more knowledge than Gandhi. He punctured Gandhi's sunlight hypothesis by explaining that only vitamin D was produced as a result of exposure to sunlight. Gandhi published McCarrison's note and thanked the doctor for his "more accurate statement." He remained skeptical of all nutritional claims, but his skepticism was tempered by a profound respect for science and data.[11]

Gandhi's nutritional approach to medicine evolved at a time of rapid change in the science of health and nutrition. As a young man, he saw firsthand what historian E. M. Collingham has called "the anachronistic nature of Anglo-Indian medicine between 1858 and 1914." The "modern medicine" practiced in India was dominated by old-fashioned doctors with old-fashioned ideas; little about it was modern. Nevertheless, British imperialists celebrated any public health achievement as the result of Western science steadily overcoming "Oriental superstition." The colonial emphasis on public health was heavily racialized, although not always in ways that divided the English from "the natives." Sometimes nutrition was used to divide Indians themselves.[12]

The British celebration of wheat and denigration of rice, for example, used a specious link between health and diet to buttress the colonial practice of divide and rule. As the wheat debate makes clear, nutrition served as a form of control and discipline, establishing the "rule of science" over Indian bodies and the Indian body politic. In rejecting Western imperialism, Gandhi at first rejected Western medicine as well. With time, however, he came to recognize the value of many Western medical practices, especially rigorous experimentation. As Gandhi's personal experiments make clear, modern nutritional science did not arrive in India as a gift from European doctors. Rather, European and Indian doctors and lay practitioners like Gandhi struggled together to understand the link between diet and health.

Despite the organic interconnectedness of his own approach to medicine, Gandhi distinguished between at least five systems of medical treatment. He defined them as follows: "(1) allopathy, (2) ayurveda, (3) unani, (4) homeopathy and (5) nature cure." The order of Gandhi's list did not indicate his own preference. It was "nature cure" that he privileged. To understand his passion for nature cure, it is first necessary to explore what he admired and did not admire about the other forms of medicine prevalent in his day. He borrowed from them all.[13]

Allopathy—also known as modern, Western, or mainstream medicine—was the response to illness Gandhi most loved to criticize. The word *allopathy* was coined by the founder of homeopathy, Samuel Hahnemann. The term *allopathic* became popular in the nineteenth century as a pejorative label for mainstream (i.e., nonhomeopathic) practice. The word comes from the Greek for "other." Whereas homeopaths treat illness by giving medicines that produce similar symptoms to those the patient is suffering, allopaths aim to remove the symptoms and thus fail to engage the underlying disease. At least, that was the argument made by Dr. Hahnemann, an argument that resonated with Gandhi. When he lambasted mainstream medicine in *Hind Swaraj*, he focused on the way in which allopathic doctors perpetuated bad behavior by curing people of the symptoms of such behavior. Rather than convince their patients to stop overeating, they offered pills to assuage indigestion.[14]

Gandhi castigated mainstream medicine for its reliance on expensive treatments and its rejection of more inexpensive indigenous remedies. Medicine was helpful, he argued, to the degree that it could help those in the greatest need. By raising costs needlessly, allopathic medicine was failing to serve the poor. Gandhi explained his criticism in 1939 in a conversation with an English missionary doctor. "Certainly good work has been done for lepers, for the blind, for sufferers from TB and other ailments," Gandhi declared, "but the help has not really touched the suffering millions of this great land." He lamented that medical treatment had been concentrated in the cities, leaving untouched "the bulk of India's population in our villages." If medicine was to help poor rural communities, it would have to be an affordable medicine that drew upon "the study of indigenous drugs and medicines." He criticized medical scientists for ignoring "indigenous talent, simply because it is not considered original or scientific." As an example, he turned to his own life. "I have had a little swelling on one foot for some days now," he explained, "which has alarmed the doctors because they feel that it is a sign denotative of commencing disintegration of the heart and kidneys." One of his colleagues, "almost an illiterate man," brought him "a green leaf" and told him that the same leaf had cured his father of the same symptom. Importantly, Gandhi did not assume that the leaf would work. Instead, he called for "an agency that can say with certainty what these herbs are and what is their quality."[15]

Gandhi's interest in natural herbs came from their low cost and wide availability. He believed all medicine should be similarly accessible. "Allopathy by itself is not expensive," he declared, "but the doctors and the chemists have made it so." His critique of medical profiteering remains all too relevant. "I wonder whether it is really a test of growth," he asked in 1925, "to find in the catalogues and in the directories of medical men that every year their sales are increasing by leaps and bounds and that the inmates in the hospitals and dispensaries are increasing." Gandhi spoke to our age as well as his own when he wondered whether increasing profits in medicine were "a sign of real progress."[16]

His belief in inexpensive natural remedies inspired his interest in India's traditional forms of medical practice, especially ayurveda. From the Sanskrit for "life science," ayurveda is an ancient form of medicine that relies on herbs and foods, as well as massage and other forms of treatment. Gandhi came to ayurveda early in life. By 1891, at the age of twenty-two, he had already developed a strong interest in the practice. That interest grew during his years in England and South Africa. Soon after returning to India from South Africa in 1915, he visited a renowned ayurvedic pharmacy and encouraged "every citizen to live his life in accordance with the principles of Ayurveda."[17]

Gandhi was not alone in publicly embracing ayurveda. In 1920, the Indian National Congress recognized "the widely prevalent and generally accepted utility of the Ayurvedic and Unani Systems of Medicine in

India." Congress delegates declared that "earnest and definite efforts should be made by the people of this country to further popularize Schools, Colleges and Hospitals for instruction and treatment in accordance with Indigenous Systems." In 1938, the Congress again publicly endorsed such "indigenous systems" of medicine. According to scholar Jean Langford, many Congress leaders praised ayurveda and unani "not because of their truth but because of their popularity and practical application, recognizing them, in a sense, as culture rather than as science." Langford explained, "Even as the Congress was campaigning for the recognition of Ayurveda as national culture, the educated elite that was its leadership was steadily losing faith in Ayurveda as a healing practice."[18]

Gandhi's opinion of ayurveda would remain positive, but his view of ayurvedic doctors changed dramatically with time. In May 1925, he was asked to lay the foundation stone at an ayurvedic college in Calcutta. He used the opportunity to denounce the state of the field. "I belong to that noble, growing, but the still small school of thought which believes more in prevention than in cure," he began. Traditional Indian medical traditions could, he felt, return medicine to a focus on prevention and on natural treatments. "There was a time," he declared, "when I used to swear by the Ayurvedic medicine and used to commend it to all my friends." That time had passed. Too many ayurvedic and unani doctors believed "they knew everything" and that "there was no disease which they could not cure."[19]

That absence of humility prevented practitioners from realizing the true potential of ayurveda. "My quarrel with the professors of [the] Ayurvedic system," Gandhi explained, "is that many of them, if not indeed a vast majority of them, are mere quacks pretending to know much more than they actually do, arrogating to themselves infallibility and [the] ability to cure all diseases." Such quacks had "no humility in them." They imputed to ayurveda "an omnipotence which it does not possess, and in so doing they have made it a stagnant system instead of a gloriously progressive science." By contrast, Gandhi praised mainstream doctors for their willingness to experiment and to be proven wrong by the data. "I know of not a single discovery or invention of any importance on the part of Ayurvedic physicians," he wrote, "as against a brilliant array of discoveries and inventions which Western physicians and surgeons boast."[20]

In his own life, Gandhi found ayurveda less effective than mainstream remedies. Nothing proved "as efficacious as quinine for malaria or iodine for simple pains." In November 1944, he became exhausted; accustomed to working long days, he found himself sapped after only a few hours. "I have grown very weak," he wrote a colleague. A doctor offered him "some pills," but he did not take them. He was "keen on getting well with the help of Ayurveda or my own methods of treatment." It is unclear precisely what treatments he sampled. His letters indicate that he experimented with *Viola cinerea*, a small herb with white flowers found in western India and known locally as *banafsha*. Whether it was the *banafsha* or another part of his treatment, something went wrong and left him weaker than he had been at the outset. "My sin in playing with Ayurveda has laid me low," Gandhi wrote a close friend and colleague. Even after suffering through this unsuccessful treatment, he did not completely discard ayurveda. He maintained his distinction between the discipline as it was practiced and the discipline itself. "I have a great regard for Ayurveda," he wrote, before adding, "My experience with those practising it has not been very good." Gandhi believed the tradition could be redeemed. "I am in search of a true practitioner of Ayurveda," he declared. A true practitioner would draw together the best practices of multiple healing traditions. "At present it is allopathy that commands enterprise, industry and knowledge," he wrote. But nothing prevented advocates of ayurveda from reinvigorating the ancient art with the best of modern science. "If Ayurveda were to take what is special in allopathy," he argued, "the latter would be left with nothing but a few drugs."[21]

To Gandhi's great dismay, the one thing that united allopathic and ayurvedic doctors was that neither group cared about the high costs of medical treatment. Gandhi called for a new approach that would "contribute to the alleviation of real suffering and make discoveries and researches in Ayurveda that will enable the poorest in the land to know and use the simple indigenous drugs." Such a practice would "teach people to learn the laws of preventing disease rather than curing them." Ayurvedic doctors too often followed their mainstream counterparts in seeking substantial profits from their labors. All forms of medicine could be exploitative—but then they were not true medicine.[22]

Gandhi endorsed mainstream medicine when it was helping those in need. In 1947, for example, he encouraged the distribution of allopathic medicines to help the thousands of refugees pouring across the new border with Pakistan. Over twenty-five thousand people were huddled at a massive refugee camp outside of Delhi. Gandhi called for "a large number of doctors" to be sent, and made clear that he had allopathic doctors in mind. Praising the physicians who were already volunteering their time to help the refugees, he stated, "They are not quacks like me."[23]

Gandhi recognized that his views on diet, nutrition, and medicine were, in his own words, "peculiar." In December 1912, he wrote an important letter to his political mentor, the renowned social reformer Gopal Krishna Gokhale. The letter aimed to solidify his relationship with the more established leader. Remarkably, his desire to earn Gokhale's respect did not prevent Gandhi from offering "one word from the quack physician." His "one word" was actually a detailed list of advice: "Ample fasting, strict adherence to two meals, entire absence of condiments of all kinds from your food, omission of pulses, tea, coffee, etc., regular taking of Kuhne baths, regular and brisk walking in the country . . . ample allowance of olive oil and acidic fruit and gradual elimination of cooked food— and you will get rid of your diabetes and add a few more years than you think to your life of service in your present body." Gandhi's advice reveals the odd duality of his relationship to nutrition—humble and self-effacing but simultaneously brimming with confidence.[24]

Gandhi's commitment to his medical beliefs complicated his relationship with his own doctors. In 1918, he fell ill and wrote a colleague, "If my sickness is still further prolonged, it will be due to my ignorance or folly, or both." He could not "ascribe any relapse to want of skill or attention of medical friends." Gandhi could not blame his doctors; they were skilled and attentive, but he was a stubborn patient, willing to accept only the advice that fit his own dietary leanings. He recognized the limits he imposed on his doctors. "They are helpless by reason of what to them are my crankisms," he explained. "But they have become part of myself and give me the greatest comfort and joy even when I am suffering excruciating pain." Gandhi's use of "they" left his meaning obscure. Was it his medical friends or his "crankisms" that had become a part of himself? Both, he might have answered. Gandhi embraced allopathic medicine while remaining committed to his own nutritional eccentricities. His blend of confidence and humility allowed such a medical pluralism. His humility also helps explain his favorite form of medicine.[25]

Although herbal remedies are often associated with premodern or non-Western societies, Gandhi developed his passion for natural medicine in London, the hub of the modern West. Most of his closest British friends shared his interest in what was then called *nature cure* or *naturopathy*. A ramshackle community of eccentric reformers, naturopaths were united by their desire to prevent and treat illness with natural methods. The definition of "natural" varied between naturopaths, but most were drawn to the use of water, earth, and diet. It matters that Gandhi first encountered nature cure in London and not in India. For him, nature cure was a universal tradition that drew upon the best medical practices from throughout the world.

Gandhi criticized naturopaths for harboring the same provincial arrogance that plagued practitioners of ayurveda. While mainstream doctors gave "a cold shoulder to naturopathy . . . the nature curists nurse a feeling of grievance against the medicos and, in spite of their very limited scientific knowledge, they make tall claims." By refusing to learn from different traditions, both mainstream doctors and naturopaths suffered from the same hubris. Gandhi's solution was for advocates of naturopathy to take up the rigorous scientific methods that had advanced mainstream medicine.[26]

Gandhi's experiments with neem demonstrate his scientific approach to natural healing. First, he learned from traditional healers which herbs were considered to have particular power. The "high merit attributed in Ayurveda" to the leaves of the neem tree sparked his interest. Next, he sought volunteers to try neem for various ailments, and experimented on himself as well. He brushed his teeth with a branch of the neem tree, and drank a concoction made of neem leaves and ginger. He then published his results alongside those of his friends and colleagues. For fever, he suggested chewing neem leaves and fasting. For blisters, he recommended boiling the leaves and then washing the blisters with the resulting water. For diarrhea, he prescribed powdered leaves. Gandhi was especially excited by the rich nutritional profile of the leaves and by the fact that neem trees grew naturally in many parts of India. "Their common use," he declared, "would enable the poor people without extra cost to take the green leaves upon which modern diet experts lay much stress." Unlike pharmaceuticals, Gandhi claimed, neem had few side effects. "That the use of the leaf produces no ill effect," he wrote, "can be stated with perfect confidence." He admitted, however, that he was "unable to say definitely what effect the taking of leaves produces on the system," and today doctors are less sanguine about the potential side effects of neem, especially for children and pregnant women.[27]

In 1935, Gandhi wrote the director of nutrition research in India, Dr. Wallace Ruddell Aykroyd, to inquire about the nutritional content of neem. In some ways, Aykroyd was the ideal person to ask. He had launched his career studying vitamin deficiency among isolated fisherfolk on the Canadian island of Newfoundland. In India, Aykroyd directed prominent studies that aimed to demonstrate how the poor could be freed from the scourge of malnutrition. Gandhi saw in Aykroyd a fellow dietary reformer focused on the needs of the poor. Would Aykroyd see Gandhi as more than a dietary faddist? Predisposed to reject traditional Indian remedies, Aykroyd decried the myth that "the diets of primitive people are superior to diets approved by science." Such a fantasy was "derivative of the eighteenth-century fiction of the happy and noble savage." Still, Gandhi asked for scientific data, and data was something Aykroyd was happy to provide. "We have analysed neem leaves in the laboratory," he wrote. "As compared with a number of other green vegetables previously investigated, they have a high nutritive value. Both mature and tender leaves are rich in protein, calcium, iron and vitamin A activity." Akroyd's letter validated Gandhi's belief in neem and his dedication to scientific rigor.[28]

Gandhi's commitment to science led him to help shutter a naturopathic hospital located in Khurja, a city not far from Delhi. The Sun and Light Hospital had been established by Shri Sharma, author of several books on naturopathy. Sharma's books offered little data in support of his claims, and his hospital likewise failed to provide the kind of evidence-based naturopathic medicine that Gandhi prized. In 1934, partly as a result of Gandhi's pressure, Sharma closed his hospital and publicly repudiated his writings. Writing about Sharma's change of heart, Gandhi reiterated his opposition to "the modern treatment of diseases" but stressed his "sneaking regard for the comparative sanity of allopaths." Allopathic doctors "do not make pretensions," he explained. "The best among them do not refuse to learn from others, and they are humble enough to own their mistakes."[29]

Gandhi's respect for modern medicine inspired him to continue his own "scientific" experiments with the healing power of fruits, vegetables, and herbs. He was drawn to tamarind, the potent fruit that lends a distinctive tartness to a variety of well-known dishes, from South Indian *sambar* to Worcestershire sauce. Tamarind interested him because of its extensive use in indigenous medicines. He experimented with the fruit as a laxative and a fever reducer, but concluded in 1935 that it was best suited as a preventive medicine, and should thus be taken regularly.[30]

If people were to consume something regularly, it would need to taste good. Gandhi recognized the need to make medicinal treatments as delicious as possible. To make neem leaves "palatable," he suggested eating them "in the form of chutney containing sufficient tamarind pulp and salt or lemon and salt." Tamarind itself he recommended eating as a jam made "with sufficient quantity of *gur*" or jaggery, the unprocessed sugar common in India. He also praised the tamarind-packed South Indian soup known as *rasam*; Gandhi asked one correspondent for his recipe and added, "You may send me medical opinion on the quality of *rasam*."[31]

Happily, some nutritional plants are already delicious. Garlic and onion, two staples throughout the world, are treasured as much for their flavor as for their nutritional value. Gandhi kept a bowl of crushed garlic on his dining table to sprinkle over his food, and celebrated the nutritional and medicinal qualities of his beloved condiment. He wrote one correspondent that garlic "helps greatly in eliminating viruses in the body" and lauded it for fostering healthy digestion and controlling blood pressure. The onion, too, offered a variety of nutritional benefits as well as a sweet, pungent flavor. Gandhi preferred both foods raw. "Garlic and onion in a raw state are strongly recommended in the West," he wrote. The virtues of the pair were also recognized by indigenous Indian traditions. "Ayurveda sings the praise of both unstintingly," Gandhi noted. Fortunately, they were widely available. "I do not know what villagers would do without garlic and onion," he declared.[32]

Gandhi prized indigenous plants, but was not opposed to introducing transplants if they might help bring proper nutrition to India's villagers. Soybeans, for example, became a favorite cause; Gandhi experimented with replacing ghee with them. The beans were soaked for several hours and then boiled. The water was kept and added to tamarind and salt to make "a very popular soup." The beans were then mixed with flaxseed oil or sesame oil and salt, "making a tasty dish." As his experiments with soy make clear, Gandhi was willing to create new culinary traditions, even while he celebrated the health benefits of old staples.[33]

Gandhi embraced soy, but his interest in other sorts of beans was tempered by concerns about digestion. He recognized that certain foods cause indigestion, and that different people have different triggers. "Dates are a fine food for a healthy stomach," he wrote, but they should be avoided by those whose digestive systems are easily upset. For indigestion, Gandhi suggested baking soda, carbonated water, or fasting—but his main recommendation was to avoid problematic foods in the first place. In addition to beans and certain fruits, milk attracted Gandhi's attention as a potential source of digestive issues. He did not know that many people lack the ability to digest the milk sugar lactose, but he recognized that those who had difficulty with milk often found relief in yogurt, which has considerably less lactose than milk and also offers friendly bacteria that contribute to digestive health. In Gandhi's words, "For some stomachs sweet curds are the best."[34]

Like yogurt, many staples of Indian cooking serve as digestion aids. While visiting Gandhi's ashram, Margaret Sanger recorded in her diary the details of a revealing meal: "Gandhiji gave me a spoonful of very bitter green puree, they were all amused at its reception & my face in getting it down. Then there was raw onions cut up in cream, one vegetable soup hot, one hot milk, flap jacks dry, a fresh orange & other vegetables & rice, really a lot of food." The "very bitter green puree" was likely *methi*, known in English as fenugreek. A common remedy for indigestion, fenugreek leaves and seeds are widely used in Indian kitchens. Even more commonplace is what Sanger described as "raw onions cut up in cream"—almost certainly *raita*, the popular Indian condiment made of yogurt, chopped onions, and various spices. Sanger noted that Gandhi himself ate a more limited meal: "goats milk & orange salad & one other vegetable puree." She explained, "He is experimenting with foods trying to find out the most economical foods for the village people & the most nourishment." While Sanger disagreed with Gandhi on many things, she approached his dietary experiments with respect and interest. As a parting gift, she left a package of figs and prunes, both of which the mahatma treasured for their ability to aid digestive regularity.[35]

Constipation was a particular specialty of doctor Gandhi. When one of his disciples fell ill, he recommended *isabgol*, an ayurvedic laxative known better as psyllium seed husk. An excellent source of soluble dietary fiber, it is the main ingredient in Metamucil and other common laxatives. Gandhi also tried cascara (bearberry), a laxative used for generations among Native Americans. His favorite source of digestive regularity was a diet rich in fruit. Eating a diverse supply of fruit was, he claimed, the best way to "keep the bowels regular." For an infection, he sometimes prescribed a juice-only diet. He especially recommended the juice of "pineapples, pomegranates, musambis, oranges and grapes." But for healthy digestion, fruit is preferable: a healthy ratio of fiber to sugar makes fruit a better choice than a high-sugar, low-fiber glass of juice.[36]

Rich with vitamins, minerals, and fiber, fruit occupied the nutritional pinnacle of Gandhi's diet. As we have seen, however, the flavors of fruit posed a dilemma. Although a delicious tamarind jam might inspire more people to reap its health benefits, its flavor could also distract from what mattered most—growing closer to God. Gandhi's religious austerity inspired him to see food as medicine. "The seeker has to have complete control over his diet," he wrote. "Whatever he eats he should eat as medicine, for the preservation of the body, never to pamper the palate." Gandhi's religious approach to diet connected personal nutrition to the larger struggle to achieve a healthy world. He understood nature cure in overtly sacred terms. "Nature cure treatment means going towards Nature, towards God," he wrote. "My quarrel with the medical profession in general is that it ignores the soul altogether."[37]

Religious beliefs complicated Gandhi's ability to link diet and nutrition. If forced to choose between religion and health, he would always choose the former. His priorities were laid bare when his vegetarianism clashed with medical opinion. In South Africa, Kasturba had to undergo an operation, and was left very thin and weak. Her doctor suggested beef broth. Gandhi refused, but the doctor secretly administered it anyway. When Gandhi learned of the surreptitious treatment, he angrily told the doctor, "I would never allow my wife to be given meat or beef, even if the denial meant her death, unless of course she desired to take it." When he asked Kasturba how she felt, she agreed to refuse any form of beef. The doctor then declined to treat her, and Gandhi removed her from the hospital. "It was drizzling and the station was some distance," he later remembered. "I was undoubtedly taking a very great risk, but I trusted in God, and proceeded with my task."[38]

Gandhi responded with equally stubborn faith when his ten-year-old son came down with typhoid and pneumonia. The family doctor explained that medicine was useless, but that "eggs and chicken broth might be given with profit." Gandhi discussed the options with his son, who agreed to refuse the eggs and chicken broth. Instead, Gandhi gave his son cold baths and "kept him on orange juice mixed with water for three days." The boy's fever persisted, going as high as 104. He became delirious. Gandhi was "haunted" by doubts, but remained firm in his beliefs. "The thread of life was in the hands of God," he later wrote. "Why not trust it to Him, and in His name go on with what I thought was the right treatment?" Gandhi left the boy with his mother, and went to walk and pray. When he returned from his walk, the fever had broken.[39]

As with his vegetarianism, Gandhi's belief in "indigenous medicine" could be extreme. He wrote a colleague treating people with fever and diarrhea that "so long as water, fire and earth are available, drugs are not necessary." He counseled sticking with nature cure even unto the death of the patients. His belief in a healthy diet sometimes led to medical exaggeration. "A balanced diet," he wrote, "gives one freedom from disease." He might have added "most of the time," but his belief in the power of diet led him to forgo his skeptical moderation.[40]

Gandhi's faith in natural medicine hinged on the relationship between mind, body, and soul. "One whose character is unworthy can never be called healthy," he proclaimed. This was more than a question of definitions. Gandhi believed in a direct causal link between morality and physical health. "The body is so closely bound to the soul," he explained, "that one whose body is pure will be pure in mind too." In fact, he declared, "a perfectly moral person alone can achieve perfect health." Being a moral person required seeing dietary reform as a way to help those in true need. After defining faith as the core of his medicine, Gandhi added that a doctor who used "such herbs as grow or can be grown in his neighbourhood purely for service of the sick and not for money may claim to be a nature-cure man." The essence of nature cure, like the essence of true faith, was serving others selflessly.[41]

Gandhi linked diet and health in pursuit of social justice, but his overemphasis on individual morality clouded his understanding of the structural inequalities that sustained poverty. Take, for example, his belief that "a perfectly moral person alone can achieve perfect health." His connection between morality and health obscured the fact that moral rectitude does not prevent a malnourished child from starving. Gandhi's belief in a moral medicine overlooked the fundamental injustice of illness. Good people fall ill, while many a cruel dictator lives long and well. As the Salt Satyagraha made clear, Gandhi was able to recognize the structural inequalities at the root of poverty. At his best, he made his diet a force for social change, not just a lesson on what to eat or not eat.

THE WOOD APPLE

In October 1935, Gandhi planned an unusual dinner party. The guests numbered just under one hundred people, mostly antipoverty activists on their way to rural villages. The highlight of the event was the food. Gandhi created the menu himself, and gave a speech carefully explaining the rationale behind every dish. The goal of the gathering was to demonstrate how to prepare a meal that was "nourishing and yet within the means of an average villager." Given the poverty of rural India, this meant dramatically limiting costs. With his dinner, Gandhi hoped to prove that a healthy meal could be prepared within the budget of India's poor.

The biggest expense was milk. Gandhi's decision to include milk is remarkable given his personal struggle to avoid consuming it. By putting milk on the menu, he prioritized the needs of the poor over his own dietary leanings. The second most expensive item was the wheat that was rolled and made into the Indian flatbreads known as chapatis. Some of Gandhi's colleagues argued that time could be saved by offering wheat porridge instead. Despite his preference for simplicity, Gandhi overruled them. He argued that chapatis could be transported more easily and made especially nutritious by using whole wheat flour and coating the dough in linseed (flaxseed) oil. Rich in nutrients including omega-3 fatty acids, the oil also had culinary benefits; it made the chapatis "both soft and crisp."

Gandhi's combination of milk and wheat would have provided plenty of protein. To be safe, he also added soybeans to the menu. He explained the soybeans as a replacement for ghee. The absence of ghee in the jails of

South Africa had enraged Gandhi. Now, he advised others to give up ghee for soybeans. He justified the substitution by declaring that the process of making ghee was "wasteful."

The fact that the majority of the budget went to protein sources should not obscure the centrality of fruits and veggies in Gandhi's meal. The menu included tomatoes and two chutneys, spiced condiments made by mixing fruits, vegetables, and spices. One of the chutneys was made with leafy greens from Gandhi's garden. The other featured *koth*, a fruit indigenous to India that is also known as wood apple or elephant apple. With a hard rind like the bark of a tree, the wood apple deserves its name. The rind must be cracked open, but the pulp inside is worth the effort. Purple and brown, with white seeds, the sticky pulp is scooped out and can be eaten plain or with sugar. Often, it is blended with coconut milk to make a beverage. The wood apple has been a part of Indian cuisine long enough to earn its own special hand pose, or *mudra*, in Indian classical dance. Gandhi proposed that it be diced and used as the base of a chutney; he added jaggery and called the result "delicious." It was not taste that made the chutney so valuable, however. Rather, it was the fact that the *koth* was "available in plenty" in that region of India, and contained a variety of health benefits. Often used as a medicine for ailments ranging from bites and stings to liver problems and indigestion, it is rich in caretenoids as well as B vitamins.

Gandhi's second chutney combined leafy greens with "some cocoanut, tamarind and salt to spice the leaves." The health benefits of coconut remain controversial, given its high fat content. Around 50 percent of the fat in coconut consists of lauric acid, a compound that raises both good and bad cholesterol, but seems to raise the good more than the bad. Regardless, the small amount of coconut Gandhi added to the chutney would not have been a health risk. The focus of the chutney was the leafy green veggies available in the garden. "Green leaves must be eaten by us," Gandhi told his guests, so that "we may get proper vitamins in our diet." Like *koth*, the green chutney was driven by accessibility for the poor. "The vegetable chosen was the cheapest available," he proclaimed, "and grows everywhere in our villages."[42]

Gandhi's meal was a success, at least on his terms. The food was nutritious and inexpensive. Each meal cost, according to Gandhi's calculations, "slightly more than six pice," approximately three or four rupees in today's currency, or roughly seven US cents. The meal was affordable even for the rural poor. Did the food taste good? Gandhi added flavorful ingredients like tamarind, and described his feast as "delicious," not a word he used lightly. More important than taste, however, was the provision of healthy food to the poor.

Harvesting wild leaves can provide one source of low-cost food, but the size of India's population convinced Gandhi that wild produce would never be enough. Existing agricultural policies did not yield sufficient fruits and vegetables for the poor, and even he found it difficult to afford a regular supply of fruit. In May 1916, he ended a raw diet because fruit cost too much. "The price of fruitarian food is prohibitive here," he wrote an old friend, "and one cannot get even dates and monkey-nuts at certain places for love or money." In April of the next year, he again ended an experiment with raw food because of the cost of fruit. "I have resumed taking cooked food from today," he wrote. "Fruit diet seems very expensive." Recognizing that the cost resulted from agricultural failures, he wrote, "There is scarcity of fruit, even in such a fertile land."[43]

To produce healthy fruits and vegetables, Gandhi became a farmer. He believed that only sustainable farming—with its cultivation of a healthy relationship between people, food, and the natural world—could provide the food necessary for everyone to live healthy lives. The more he learned from the struggles of poor farmers, the more he realized that the distribution of food was as important as its production. His romantic vision of farming collided with the brutal realities of rural India, forcing him to rethink many of his most basic assumptions about his society and himself.

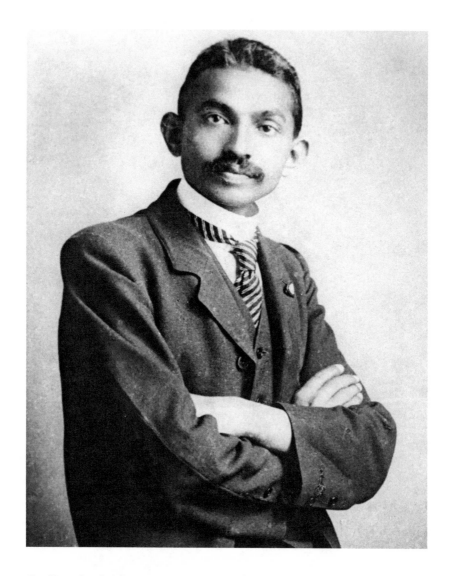

Gandhi in South Africa in 1906. A committed vegetarian with an interest in raw food, he cut salt from his diet, vowed to never drink milk, and connected his experiments with food to his early efforts with nonviolent civil disobedience. Courtesy of Wikimedia Commons.

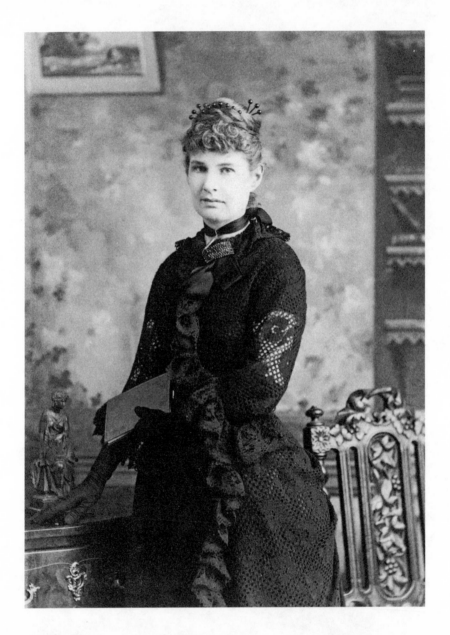

Anna Kingsford, one of the first English women to receive a medical degree, and the author of a best-selling defense of vegetarianism, *The Perfect Way in Diet*. In South Africa, Gandhi sold copies of Kingsford's book and repeatedly quoted her in support of vegetarianism. Courtesy of Wikimedia Commons.

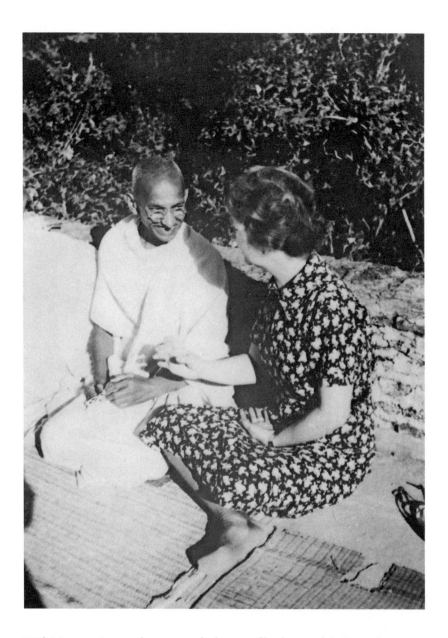

With Margaret Sanger, the renowned advocate of birth control, in December 1935.
In order to distinguish between love and lust, Gandhi compared eating chocolate
to having sex. Sanger was intrigued by Gandhi's dietary experiments, but rejected
his views on sex and chocolate. Courtesy of the Library of Congress.

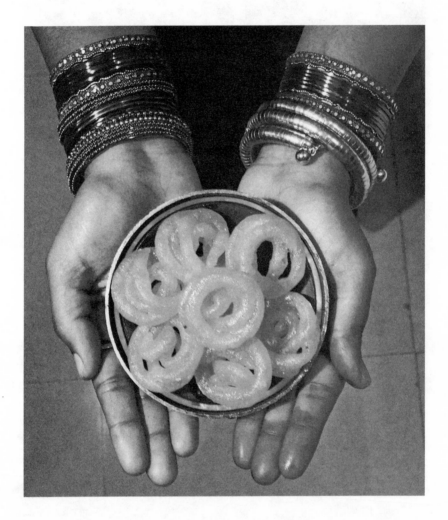

"Is it not better," Gandhi wrote in 1934, "that one who daily eats *jalebi* in his imagination should eat the real thing and know the wisdom or folly of doing so?" Made with a wheat flour known as *maida*, *jalebi* are fried, soaked in syrup, and sometimes flavored with lime juice or rose water. As a young man, Gandhi recommended that Indian travelers carry *jalebi* to remind them of home; later, however, he used the sweet to symbolize temptation. Black and white derivative of photo by Avanthika Duraiswamy licensed under CC-BY-SA-4.0, Wikimedia Commons.

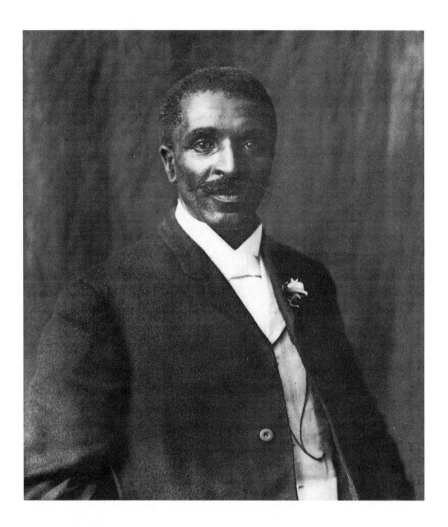

The renowned scientist George Washington Carver in 1906. In the late 1930s, Carver developed a peanut milk that Gandhi hoped would allow him to become vegan. Although Gandhi praised Carver as a "genius," the peanut milk failed to end Gandhi's dependence on goat's milk. Courtesy of the Library of Congress.

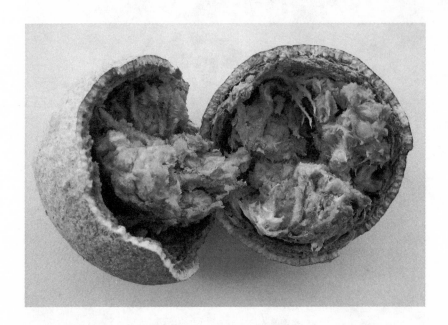

The wood apple, a fruit indigenous to India, known to Gandhi as *koth*. In October 1935, Gandhi included wood apple in a model menu he designed to demonstrate that a nourishing meal could be prepared within the budget of India's poor. The fruit was plentiful in much of rural India, and thus offered an affordable source of nutrition. The name *wood apple* can refer to two distinct fruit trees, *Aegle marmelos* (often known in Hindi as *bael*) and *Limonia acidissima* (featured here). Courtesy of Seisfeldt at Wikimedia Commons.

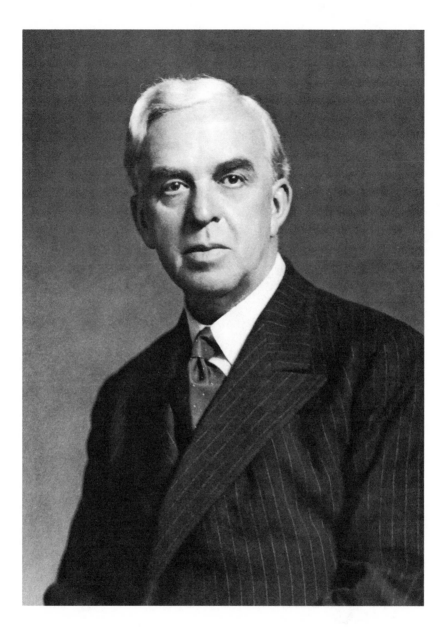

Robert McCarrison, head of nutritional research in India and Gandhi's most prominent nutritional antagonist, pictured in April 1935. McCarrison lectured Gandhi on the need for meat (the mahatma remained unconvinced) and corrected Gandhi's views on vitamin D. But the two men agreed on the value of fresh, unprocessed food and the importance of organic agriculture. McCarrison became one of the few non-Indian members of the advisory board of the All-India Village Industries Association, the organization Gandhi founded to advance his vision of sustainable rural development. © National Portrait Gallery, London.

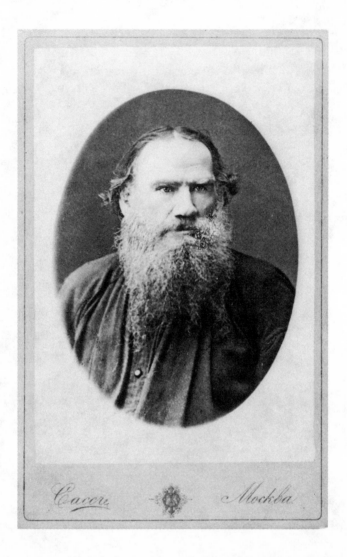

Leo Tolstoy, renowned writer, vegetarian, and advocate of nonviolence, photo-graphed sometime between 1880 and 1886. Gandhi's nonviolence was shaped by vegetarian activists like Tolstoy. The two men corresponded, and Gandhi named one of his model communities Tolstoy Farm. "He has given up all his vices," Gandhi wrote of Tolstoy, "eats very simple food and has it in him no longer to hurt any living being by thought, word or deed." Courtesy of the Library of Congress.

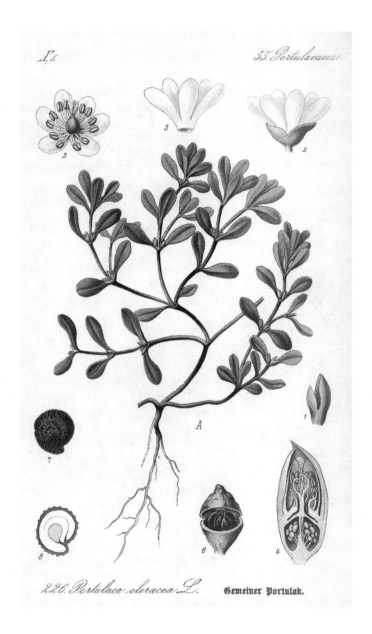

226. *Portulaca oleracea L.* Gemeiner Portulak.

Purslane (*Portulaca oleracea*), a common "weed" in many parts of the world, known to Gandhi as *luni*. Purslane offers vitamins A, B, and C, some protein, and more omega-3 fatty acids than almost any other vegetable source. Its combination of nutrition and availability fueled Gandhi's belief that wild foods could provide vital nutrients for the rural poor. From Otto Wilhelm Thomé, *Flora von Deutschland, Österreich und der Schweiz in Wort und Bild für Schule und Haus* (Gera-Untermhaus: F. E. Köhler, 1885).

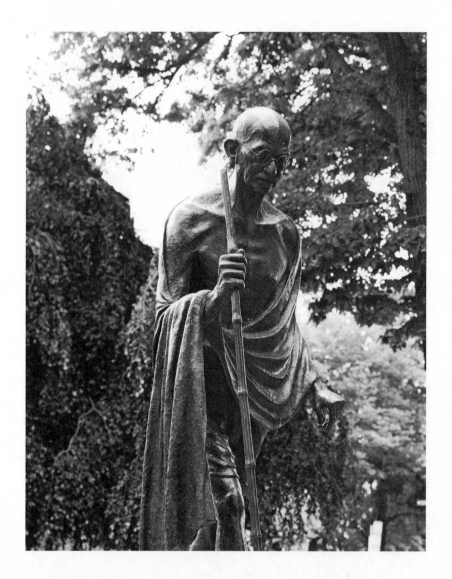

Photograph by Carol M. Highsmith of a statue of Gandhi created by Gautam
Pal, dedicated in 2000, and located near the Indian embassy in Washington, DC.
Gandhi's body, a global icon that symbolizes humility and nonviolence, was shaped
by a lifetime of experiments with food and nutrition. Despite the public attention
his body received, and his obsession with diet, Gandhi remained uninterested in the
connection between what he ate and how he looked. Photo courtesy of the Carol M.
Highsmith Archive, Library of Congress, Prints and Photographs Division.

CHAPTER 6

Farming

Your diet should contain some greens. You should grow them in
your own backyard.

GANDHI, 1926

I N OCTOBER 1919, GANDHI DECLARED IN BOMBAY, "I WANT TO BE
known as a farmer and a weaver." Gandhi the weaver has been immor-
talized in images: the bespectacled mahatma with his iconic spinning
wheel. Gandhi the farmer, by contrast, has been largely forgotten. Gandhi began farming as a young man in South Africa, and continued to
grow his own fruits and vegetables throughout his life. Farming embodied many of his most deeply held ideals—self-reliance, sustainability,
economy, and connection to nature. Ultimately, it was his passion for
food that inspired his farming. Gandhi respected the ecology in which all
things grow: the richer the soil, the deeper the roots, the stronger the
plant. In the words of the poet Wendell Berry, "Eating is an agricultural
act." By connecting his diet to his farming, Gandhi recognized the relationship between the land and human civilization—as well as the many
ways human beings have distorted that relationship.[1]

Despite his devotion to farming, Gandhi dedicated only a small
amount of his time to growing crops. He had the resources to make farming a hobby rather than the foundation of his livelihood and, like many
amateurs, he romanticized farming. He was inspired by Sir Henry Maine,
a renowned historian and jurist, who served as vice-chancellor of the

University of Calcutta. In books and public lectures, Maine popularized an image of the ancient Indian village as a self-sustaining agricultural paradise, a vision that Gandhi adopted and made his own. Importantly, Gandhi's utopian vision of the Indian village did not prevent him from recognizing the problems that confronted villagers. He bemoaned the lack of "practical knowledge" that led to "ignorant superstition," and he decried the absence of sanitation that left many villages little more than "muck-heaps." Still, he placed great hope in the future of the village as the center of a healthier and more just India.[2]

In addition to Henry Maine, Gandhi was influenced by John Ruskin, who rejected modern industrial society in favor of an idealized pastoral utopia. In 1904, one of Gandhi's vegetarian friends gave him a copy of Ruskin's *Unto This Last*. He later remembered, "I determined to change my life in accordance with the ideals of the book." Three of Ruskin's ideals were especially important:

1. That the good of the individual is contained in the good of all.
2. That a lawyer's work has the same value as the barber's in as much as all have the same right of earning their livelihood from their work.
3. That a life of labour, i.e., the life of the tiller of the soil and the handicraftsman is the life worth living.

Of these ideals, the third struck Gandhi with special force. The full value of tilling the soil "had never occurred" to him. In 1908, he translated *Unto This Last* into Gujarati and coined a new word to serve as its title: *sarvodaya*, a compound of *sarva* (all) and *udaya* (uplift), or as Gandhi himself explained it, "the welfare of all."[3]

Sarvodaya depended on agriculture. Even as his own farming became marginalized by other pursuits, Gandhi's interest in rural development grew stronger. His understanding of rural poverty was hampered by his romantic vision of farming as well as by his political dependence on large landowners. A vast chasm separated his garden from the fields of rural India. But he worked to close that divide by confronting the poverty of farmers and empowering them to regain control of their own lives. Importantly, his focus was not limited to India. He grappled with how the global food system could be rendered more humane and more equitable. His efforts to achieve rural sustainability remain relevant at a time in which futures markets in New York dictate the price of corn in rural Mexico, and millions of farmers struggle to get enough to eat.[4]

HOME ECONOMICS

In 1922, Gandhi wrote a story about farming called "The Field and the Vadi"—a *vadi* being a garden dedicated to fruits and vegetables. The story took the form of a conversation between a mother and a child. The mother asked, "Do you know what crops grow in our village?" "Yes, mother," the child replied, "wheat, gram, *bajra, tuvar, jowar*, etc., according to the season." Pearl millet (*bajra*), pigeon pea (*tuvar*), sorghum (*jowar*)—this child knew her grains. And well she should, Gandhi implied. Just as our bodies require a varied diet, so farmers have learned the merits of agricultural diversity. Some plants, like millet and sorghum, are drought resistant; some provide nitrogen for the soil; others repel pesky bugs. By planting a variety of crops, farmers minimize their reliance on synthetic fertilizers and pesticides. For a poor farmer in India, there is an additional reason to cultivate diverse crops: with limited access to markets, growing a variety of foods is the best way to eat a variety of foods.[5]

Gandhi's lesson for children linked agricultural diversity to collective social action. Despite the range of grains grown in her village, the child lectured her mother that they ought to grow more. "The absence of a *vadi* near the village is felt very badly," she declared. A neighboring village had neem trees, tamarind trees, mango trees, jujube plants, and a vegetable *vadi* boasting "beans, brinjals, fenugreek, java radish, lady's fingers, radishes and so on." "Ours is a poor village," the mother explained. "There is no unity among the residents, so the people rest content with the crops that grow in our fields." Without collective action, Gandhi suggested, India's food system would remain unjust and unhealthy.[6]

We eat what we can eat, what is available and affordable. Gandhi recognized the relationship between diet and food availability. In an 1893 letter from South Africa, he told readers of the *Vegetarian* that he had convinced his landlady to stop eating meat. He worried, however, that her vegetarianism would not last. "Proper vegetables cannot be had here," he explained. Without a regular supply of affordable fruits and vegetables, how could anyone remain vegetarian? To remedy the situation, he asked for a "vegetarian gardener."[7]

While he recognized that "all men are not going to be farmers," Gandhi encouraged everyone to plant a small garden. From Yeravda jail, he wrote a friend, "If you settle down at one place, why should you not grow in the yard some vegetables which would take only a short time to grow?" Gandhi believed gardening built character. Perhaps the most famous quote attributed to the mahatma speaks to the centrality of personal growth to his philosophy: "Be the change you want to see in the world." Gandhi never said those words, but he expressed a similar sentiment in more organic terms when he declared, "A creeper yielding bitter fruit will never bear jasmines and the *palasha* will not yield mangoes." The *palasha*, also known as "flame of the forest" or "bastard teak," is a beautiful tree with deep red flowers, widely used for medicinal purposes in India. By comparing it to a mango tree, Gandhi did not mean to say that one plant is better than another or, by extension, that one way of life is better than another. In its own way, the *palasha* was as useful as the mango. Gandhi's point was that if we are to live up to our own ambitions, we must learn to change not just what we do, but who we are. His reference to the *palasha* came in an editorial he published in South Africa in 1907. At that time, the Indian community in South Africa was fighting for its rights against a racist government. By juxtaposing the *palasha* and the mango, Gandhi encouraged his readers to come together as a community and to grow as individuals in order to defend their rights. It is fitting that he used botanical metaphors to stress that each of us must change if we are to change the world. He believed that gardening helped him embody his values.[8]

One of Gandhi's most treasured values—frugality—played a central role in inspiring his love of gardens. His diet could "effect considerable economy" because he was able to grow his own vegetables. He calculated that his homegrown diet cost a third of what he would spend if he bought his produce. "Instead of raisins and dates," he wrote, "I eat daily seven or eight tomatoes, four or five big-sized, baked sweet potatoes and about six spoons of cabbage or any other vegetable that is available." What was available did not depend on the local market. "I get the vegetables from what grows in the garden here," he explained.[9]

Frugality drove Gandhi's love for gardens, but that love went well beyond economy. He encouraged members of his ashram to grow vegetables "even if it is more expensive to do so than to buy them." *Swaraj* required self-sustainability in all things basic to survival, and nothing was more basic than food. At times, self-sufficiency demanded flexibility. "When no vegetable can be served," Gandhi wrote, "I would have tamarind fruits plucked from the trees and serve chutney prepared from their pulp crushed with salt." As the ashram garden demonstrated, growing a diverse supply of fresh fruits and vegetables is a form of nutritional insurance.[10]

A diverse garden is an organic library, offering knowledge as well as nutrition. Gardening offered Gandhi another way to know his food, as well as medicinal plants like neem and the palm starch known as sago, a common ingredient in ayurvedic treatments. Gandhi encouraged his friends and followers to cultivate medicinal plants like neem and sago, as well as fruits, vegetables, and other staples. "Intensify your interest in agriculture," he advised one colleague. While the products of agriculture were crucial for the development of society, the process of agriculture was equally vital for human development.[11]

Gandhi believed that growing food offered an opportunity to combine physical and mental exercise. "Just as food is necessary for the mind as much as for bones and flesh, so also is exercise necessary both for body and mind," he wrote in 1913. "Real exercise is that which trains, continuously, both mind and body alike." Farming was the ideal form of such "real exercise." In his own experience, Gandhi benefited from the healthfulness of farming, but his emphasis on such benefits led him to overlook the hardships that many farmers faced. His praise of the mental challenges of farming ignored the possibility that such challenges would be stressful. According to Gandhi, the farmer "must be able to test the nature of his soil, must watch changes of weather, must know how to manipulate his plough skillfully and be generally familiar with the movements of the stars, the sun and the moon." Such mental demands, coupled with the physical requirements of farming, struck him as the ideal exercise for mind and body. But these challenges could just as readily lead to stress and exhaustion. Among the poorest members of Indian society, farmers often live at the whim of forces beyond their control. Gandhi's praise of the rural lifestyle reveals the gap between his romantic conception of village life and the reality of rural exploitation—in his day as well as our own.[12]

That gap is particularly prominent in Gandhi's relationship with the farmer's greatest friend and greatest foe—the sun. In addition to providing exercise and fresh air, gardening allowed Gandhi to benefit from the sun's healing powers. He did not have to worry about getting enough vitamin D. In addition to gardening, he indulged regularly in what he called "a sun bath." Meanwhile, many farmers in India struggled to stay out of the sun, and were forced to work long hours in unrelenting heat.[13]

Gandhi often failed to recognize the chasm that separated his experiments with agriculture from the reality confronting many of India's poorest farmers. In 1910, he republished a popular poem often included in textbooks for elementary school students. The poem began:

> O tiller of the soil,
> Rightly they call you father of the world;
> You, and you alone, provide
> For all mankind.

The poem praised farmers for "braving heat and rain," but failed to recognize the brutal conditions many farmers faced. "Robust of health" and full of "contentment," Gandhi's ideal farmers dwelled in a fantasy land, unknown to the landless laborers that continue to do the bulk of farm labor in many parts of the world. Gandhi's conception of farming seems absurd in light of the inequalities of the modern agricultural system. Why did he romanticize a profession that entails long hours of brutal work, often without access to clean water or decent food?[14]

His own experience as a part-time farmer explains some of Gandhi's utopian fantasies, but the real source of those fantasies was his hope for the future. He dreamed of a society in which farming would bring health and contentment to everyone—including the farmer—and he believed that the virtues of farming were crucial to achieving such a society. Selfless service was the most important of those virtues. "Of course the farmer is the father of the world," he wrote, "but it is his greatness that he is not aware of the fact." Gandhi hoped that the selfless service of the farmer could cut through materialism, greed, and inequality. "If the farmer is indeed a father and if his profession is indeed the highest," he asked, "why are we busy padding ourselves with heaps of clothes? Why do we grind the poor under our heels to extort the last farthing from them?"[15]

Gandhi struggled to change a system in which those who grew food did not get enough to eat. In India, he wrote in 1942, fruits and vegetables were "generally considered to be delicacies meant for the city people." In the villages, he lamented, "fresh vegetables are a rarity and in most places fruit is also not available." He saw a revolution in farming as the best way to heal the broken relationship between city and countryside.[16]

Gandhi's idealized notion of farming did not prevent him from denouncing the inequality that continues to mark the global food system. Indeed, he used his vision of an agricultural utopia to highlight the injustice of the so-called civilized world. His goal was not just to increase the amount of food available, but to make sure that all resources were shared fairly, that no one went without food to eat. He was not opposed to using the most recent science to increase agricultural output, but his focus remained on ensuring equal access, especially to fresh fruits and vegetables. He recognized that the supply of healthy food depends on food security, food equality, and ultimately food democracy.[17]

ANTI-IMPERIAL AGRICULTURE

Gandhi knew that individual gardens would not end poverty. Many poor people lack the space and money to begin a garden. In an urbanized world, small-scale gardens cannot meet the vast demand for food. Small farms, on the other hand, might be able to meet that demand, especially if they work together.

Take the case of milk cooperatives. "Milk is an essential article of diet," Gandhi told village-level volunteers in 1935. "It ought to be considered a shame that milk is not available in many of our villages." As we have seen, Gandhi's reevaluation of milk was remarkable; something he struggled to avoid became "an essential article of diet." In the mid-1940s, a group of farmers in Gandhi's home state of Gujarat offered their own dramatic change of course; they reinvented how their milk was processed and sold. At the time, farmers traveled long distances to sell to the only dairy in the region that processed and distributed milk. One of Gandhi's closest colleagues, Vallabhbhai Patel, suggested that the farmers create a collaborative. They could share the costs of processing the milk and the profits of selling it and thus cut out the middlemen. The cooperative those farmers formed, known as Amul, is now one of India's largest dairy producers. Owned by three million farmers, Amul demonstrates the power of agricultural cooperatives. Its farmer-owners helped spark a "white revolution" that increased dramatically the supply of milk to India's villages.[18]

Agricultural cooperatives can help many farmers, but as Gandhi was keenly aware, the poverty in India's villages points to a larger challenge confronting modern society—the challenge of scarcity in the midst of abundance. The lack of produce in villages full of farmers reveals a fundamental weakness of the political and economic order. Gandhi deemed the shortage of fresh produce "a slur on the administration of India." He encouraged all Indians to "grow plenty of green vegetables," but he also demanded that the government support better agricultural policies that would help end inequality itself.[19]

During his years in South Africa, Gandhi learned to associate food availability with politics, to see in the starving man the work of imperial neglect. His changing views on famine reveal his growing understanding of the politics of diet. In 1897, a twenty-eight-year-old Gandhi responded to impending famine in India by praising the British Empire. He noted that famines "as a rule" occurred in India "every four years," and recognized the brutality of mass starvation. "Children are snatched from their mothers," he wrote, "wives from their husbands." Still, he depicted the government as a beneficial force. As a result of famine, he wrote, "Whole tracts are devastated, and this in spite of the precautions taken by a most benevolent Government." Gandhi failed to consider whether "a most benevolent Government" might be responsible for the economic conditions in which famine recurred every four years.[20]

Gandhi praised the British in an effort to cajole them into taking action. "Whether it be in the United Kingdom or in the Colonies," he wrote, "I am sure British philanthropy will assert itself, as it has on previous occasions, on behalf of suffering humanity." Such a statement, while perhaps justifiable as a form of gentle pressure, also reveals that Gandhi had yet to become an anti-imperial radical. Writing in 1900, he went so far as to hope that the famine might help strengthen the empire. If war united "the various parts of the mighty Empire to which it is our pride to belong," he wrote, perhaps famine might "be the means of forging another link in the chain that ties all together."[21]

With time, Gandhi would learn to see the imperial "chain that ties all together" as a form of slavery—a chain of bondage he would vow to break. His early belief in the benevolence of the British Empire should not obscure, however, the fact that he recognized how inequalities of food bound the world together. He called for a compassionate response that stretched across distance and national borders. He focused more on charity than on anti-imperial protest. Nevertheless, he highlighted perhaps the most important reason that hunger persists in a world of plenty—the widespread ability of human beings to ignore the suffering of others.

Gandhi recognized that the anonymity of distance limited the noble intentions of his countrymen. "If you saw a man dying at your door of hunger," he wrote, "you would give all you may have to satisfy the hunger of that dying man." In the case of famine, he continued, "the only difference is that millions are dying of hunger far away from you." Distance was no excuse for inaction in the face of suffering—and neither should the seeming impotence of the individual limit action. Gandhi rejected the excuse "that what you may give will be of no use." "It is the drops that make the ocean," he declared. It is "the duty of every one of us to give the utmost we can."[22]

In a world marred by inequality, charity could only do so much. Ultimately, Gandhi did not want to help the poor; he wanted to end poverty. Over time, he developed a deeper understanding of the link between famine and imperialism. "India suffers from starvation because there is dearth not of grain," he explained, "but of purchasing power." The absence of purchasing power was, in turn, a direct result of the economic structures of British rule. In the wake of repeated famines, the British claim to good governance had become "sheer pretence and mockery." Recognizing famine as a result of empire inspired Gandhi to demand India's freedom. "In the name of justice and for the good of humanity," he declared, "India must be given home rule."[23]

In his quest to feed the starving, Gandhi moved from appealing to British philanthropy to indicting the imperial system that created famines. His critique of social inequality was complicated by his belief in the dignity of labor. "To a people famishing and idle," he wrote, "the only acceptable form in which God can dare appear is work and the promise of food as wages." The poor should not be given food; "they can earn it only by the sweat of their brow," he asserted. Despite his glorification of labor,

Gandhi recognized the injustice of a world in which some worked endlessly and starved while others ate lavishly without doing any work at all. "God created man to work for his food," and "those who ate without work were thieves." The inequality of Indian society led directly to foreign rule. India was so divided, Gandhi asked, "Is it any wonder if India has become one vast prison?"[24]

Gandhi's understanding of famine was put to the test by one of the most brutal holocausts of the twentieth century. In 1943 and 1944, several million people starved to death in Bengal. As with most famines, natural disasters played a role in the calamity, but so did government policy. In the midst of the Second World War, the colonial government was focused on supplying the Allied war machine. At the height of the famine, grain flowed out of Bengal to feed soldiers. Gandhi was convinced "that the famine was man-made and not a natural calamity." He blamed the British government for the disaster, and said so bluntly to the governor of Bengal.[25]

A few years later, Gandhi had the opportunity to help prevent another mass starvation. After learning from a colleague that potato farmers could not access seed plants, he wrote the governor to urge immediate action. The government used emergency powers to confiscate seed potatoes, which were distributed to farmers just in time to be planted. Gandhi had learned that farming was as political as it was natural. To ensure a healthy food supply, the government needed to be guarded as closely as the crops themselves.[26]

Gandhi's connection between food supply and politics went well beyond preventing famine. In South Africa, he encouraged his readers to take up agriculture, but stressed that they would first have to discard their racial prejudices. "If a few men could be induced to turn their attention from the Johannesburg gold to the quieter method of earning money by cultivation, and to get rid of their colour prejudice," he wrote, "there is no doubt that every variety of vegetable and fruit could be grown in Natal." White South Africans would need to let go of "colour prejudice" in order to learn from other South Africans, regardless of their color, who had experience tilling the soil. While Gandhi focused primarily on the talents of his fellow Indians, his own life story demonstrates his debt to the rich agricultural wisdom of black South Africans.[27]

As we have seen, Gandhi's relationship to rural development was shaped by John Langalibalele Dube. In 1900, Dube opened the Zulu

Christian Industrial School on the outskirts of Durban. Students at Dube's school, later renamed the Ohlange Institute, learned technical skills and the importance of hard work, self-improvement, and community solidarity. A few years after Dube founded his school, Gandhi opened his own model community, the Phoenix Settlement, just a few miles from the Ohlange Institute. The two model communities remained on good terms. In November 1912 one of Gandhi's mentors, the Indian National Congress leader and prominent social worker Gopal Krishna Gokhale, came to South Africa and met Dube at the Ohlange Institute. Discussing his meeting with Gokhale in his newspaper *Ilanga*, Dube wrote, "We have seen and heard a great man whose knowledge is equal to that of the foremost statesmen of our day, and he is a black man." A close associate of Gandhi, the English priest C. F. Andrews, later remembered finding at Gandhi's house "a young Zulu Christian lady treated by Gandhi as his own daughter from the Rev. Mr. Dubay's Mission just outside his own religious centre." With some hyperbole, but not without cause, Andrews proclaimed, "So close were they all together in that settlement that it made no difference that they belonged to different races for they were one in heart and love." Like mealie pap, farming had challenged Gandhi's views on race and class and helped him grow as a human being. The more he valued working on the land, the more he discarded his early belief in the superiority of certain kinds of "civilization." True civilization, he realized, came from honest work—and no work was more important than farming.[28]

Gandhi founded the Phoenix Settlement in 1904. Like John Dube, he aimed to create a self-sustaining community that would serve as a model for society. To maximize the social impact of his experiment, he publicized the farm as widely as possible. One of the first additions to the settlement was a printing press, hauled to the remote site by some sixty-four oxen. The press was necessary; Gandhi used it to produce his newspaper *Indian Opinion*, with which he launched a frontal assault on a society divided by race and class. With Phoenix as a home base, he attacked injustice and modeled the world he hoped to build.[29]

Agriculture was the foundation of this experiment in communal living. A river ran through the hundred-acre settlement, watering an assortment of fruit trees and vegetable gardens. In addition to food, those gardens provided the opportunity to work in what Gandhi saw as the most ennobling profession. "Agriculture is the true occupation of man," he wrote. By contrast, industrialization made it so that "a few can wallow in riches by exploiting the helplessness and poverty of the many." Gandhi located his critique of food inequality within a larger struggle against the social and political hierarchies of his time. Even as he dedicated his life to changing society, he intensified his efforts to create a rural utopia separate from society.[30]

In 1910, he established his second agrarian community, Tolstoy Farm, in the rural hinterland of Johannesburg. As we have seen, Gandhi was drawn to Tolstoy's vegetarianism and radical compassion. "He has given up all his vices," Gandhi wrote in 1905, "eats very simple food and has it in him no longer to hurt any living being by thought, word or deed."[31]

In 1909, Gandhi summoned the courage to write Tolstoy directly. His letter, sent from the Westminster Palace Hotel in London, reveals his humility as well as his audacity. He denounced "the prejudice against colour" as an assault on "the spirit of true religion," and explained that Tolstoy's writings had inspired him to embrace "the doctrine of non-resistance to evil." Tolstoy had written an open letter attacking the rise of revolutionary violence in India. Gandhi praised the letter, and asked permission to have twenty thousand copies printed and distributed. As if that were not sufficiently bold, he suggested that Tolstoy amend his concluding paragraph to remove a critique of reincarnation. "Reincarnation or transmigration is a cherished belief with millions in India," Gandhi explained. "My object in writing this is not to convince you of the truth of the doctrine," he added; he hoped only that the reference to reincarnation be deleted out of respect for Hindu opinion.[32]

Tolstoy responded a week later. He expressed "great pleasure" at reading Gandhi's note, and praised the South African struggle as a "fight between gentleness and brutality, between humility and love on one side, and conceit and violence on the other." In regard to reincarnation, Tolstoy modeled the tolerant pluralism that he and Gandhi shared. "As it appears to me," he explained, "the belief in a re-birth will never be able to strike such deep roots in and restrain mankind as the belief in the immortality of the soul and the faith in divine truth and love." His personal belief did not prevent him from respecting the views of others. "Of course I would accommodate you," he told Gandhi, "if you so desire, to delete those passages in question." Gandhi had offered to pay Tolstoy for the right to publish his writings. Tolstoy waved aside such financial considerations. "The question regarding monetary payment of Royalty," he explained, "should not at all be allowed to appear in religious undertakings."[33]

Gandhi moved quickly to solidify Tolstoy's support for the struggle in South Africa. Once again, he blended modesty with ambitious self-promotion. He sent a biography of himself written by an admiring friend, and told Tolstoy that "this struggle of the Indians in the Transvaal is the greatest of modern times." A few months later, Gandhi sent a copy of *Hind Swaraj*. Tolstoy appreciated Gandhi's emphasis on nonviolence, but his anticolonial nationalism, equally central to *Hind Swaraj*, clashed with Tolstoy's internationalism. Tolstoy wrote privately that Gandhi's "Hindu patriotism . . . spoils everything." That assessment did not prevent him from continuing his warm correspondence with Gandhi or praising his book. Tolstoy told Gandhi, "I think the question you have therein dealt with is important not only for Indians, but for the whole of mankind."[34]

The question Tolstoy had in mind was how to overcome injustice nonviolently. In September 1910, he wrote Gandhi that "what one calls nonresistance, is in reality nothing else but the discipline of love." The discipline of love was, for Tolstoy, profoundly Christian. His religious differences with Gandhi might have served as a wedge between the two men. Instead, their mutual tolerance allowed them to see beyond their differences to their shared values. Both men understood nonviolence in fundamentally religious terms—and as a radical force. "Either it must be admitted that we do not recognise any discipline, religious or moral, and that we are guided in the organisation of life only by the law of force," Tolstoy wrote Gandhi, "or that all the taxes that we exact by force, the judicial and police organisations and, above all, the army must be abolished." Abolishing taxes, the courts, the police, and the army—this was not a conservative strategy. Tolstoy embraced revolutionary nonviolence, and he recognized Gandhi's struggle in South Africa as a model. Gandhi was equally appreciative of Tolstoy's expansive nonviolence. In his introduction to Tolstoy's "Letter to a Hindu," Gandhi declared, "Tolstoy's life has been devoted to replacing the method of violence for removing tyranny or securing reform by the method of nonresistance to evil."[35]

Gandhi told Tolstoy about the naming of Tolstoy Farm, and forwarded copies of *Indian Opinion* that discussed the community. As Gandhi made clear, the farm embodied many of the values that he and Tolstoy shared. Their religious tolerance, for example, found expression in the diversity of the residents: Hindus, Muslims, Parsis, and Christians. The majority, about forty, were men; five women and some thirty children lived at the farm. Together, the residents aimed to demonstrate the nonviolence and self-reliance that Tolstoy and Gandhi associated with rural living at its best.

Over a thousand acres, the farm boasted hundreds of fruit trees that produced almonds, walnuts, apricots, peaches, and figs. In his book *Satyagraha in South Africa*, Gandhi celebrated the land's natural abundance. "Upon the Farm," he remembered, "oranges, apricots and plums grew in such abundance that during the season the Satyagrahis could have their fill of the fruit and yet have a surplus besides." The community was a model of sustainability. Water was transported manually from a nearby spring. Wastewater was gathered in buckets and used to water the trees. A compost system turned food waste and human waste into fertile manure. Residents made their own sandals. It was, in Gandhi's words, "a busy hive of industry."[36]

Economy was a priority. Rather than waste money on train fare, residents walked over twenty miles to get to Johannesburg. "The general practice," Gandhi explained, "was that the sojourner should rise at two o'clock and start at half past two." The journey took six to seven hours. Residents carried their food with them so as to avoid spending any money in the city. Their simple picnics included homemade whole wheat bread, peanut butter, and orange marmalade. The peanut butter was made by roasting and grinding the peanuts and was, Gandhi proudly recorded, "four times cheaper than ordinary butter."[37]

The food at Tolstoy Farm epitomized Gandhi's diet. For breakfast, bread and coffee were served; both were made from roasted wheat. The farm had an iron hand mill to grind the wheat. "The bread is made at home," Gandhi stressed, "without the use of yeast." For lunch, residents ate rice, lentils, and more whole wheat bread served "with home-made jam prepared from oranges growing on the farm." Dinner consisted of porridge, bread, and jam. For snacks, dried fruit and peanuts were sometimes available, but fresh fruit and vegetables were more common. Everyone ate together, using simple wooden bowls they made themselves.[38]

The communal nature of their meals reinforced the unity of the residents, but also posed challenges to that unity. Several of the Christians and Muslims were meat eaters before they arrived at Tolstoy Farm. Gandhi wanted all the food to be vegetarian, but did not feel justified in banning meat altogether. Instead, he explained the low cost of vegetarian cuisine as well as his own "deep-rooted sentiment in the matter." After hearing Gandhi's appeal, the meat eaters agreed to remain vegetarian during their time at the farm. Vegetarianism was only one way in which food helped overcome religious divisions. Many of the Hindu residents observed fasts on a regular basis. When Ramadan arrived, many joined their Muslim friends in avoiding food during daylight hours.[39]

The religious unity of the residents stands in contrast to the persistent racial divisions that marked the relationship between Tolstoy Farm and the surrounding communities of black South Africans. In building the farm, Gandhi employed black labor without inviting any black South Africans to join as members of the community. A report printed in Gandhi's newspaper reveals the racial divide at Tolstoy Farm. The report described the construction of the farm in starkly racial terms: "Mr. Chinan, Mr. Kuppusamy Naidoo, Mr. Manilal Gandhi and Mr. Gandhi have been working at stone-rolling side by side with the Kaffirs." While the Indians were recognized by name, the black South Africans remained anonymous "Kaffirs." Gandhi was aware that racial injustice defined land ownership in South Africa. "The Negroes alone are original inhabitants of this land," he wrote in 1910. "The whites," he explained, "have occupied the country forcibly and appropriated it to themselves." By contrast, he continued, "We have not seized the land from [the black South Africans] by force; we live here with their goodwill." Gandhi's history was misleading; he failed to acknowledge the degree to which Indian traders benefited from a system based on the racial exclusion of blacks. Instead of encouraging his Indian readers to help black South Africans regain their land, he defended the land rights of Indians. "We think we have as much right to be in this land as the whites have," he concluded. Gandhi's claims came at a time when racist laws targeted Indians. He aimed to support an immigrant community under attack by white supremacists.

Nevertheless, his comments reveal the limits of his solidarity with black South Africans.[40]

Over the course of his time in South Africa, Gandhi would move toward racial inclusivity—inspired, in part, by his experiences as a farmer. It matters that the black South Africans who helped build Tolstoy Farm remained anonymous, but it also matters that Gandhi and his colleagues worked "side by side" with those often deemed inferior. At Tolstoy Farm, everyone worked. "Here we insisted that we should not have any servants," Gandhi explained. In 1910, he drafted a remarkable contract with his close friend Hermann Kallenbach. A Jewish architect born in Germany, Kallenbach had become one of his most trusted confidantes. It was Kallenbach who provided the money to buy Tolstoy Farm, and who suggested naming it after Tolstoy. Like Tolstoy, Gandhi and Kallenbach believed in the redemptive power of labor, especially the kind of labor demanded on a farm. Their contract made clear that "the primary object of going to the Farm so far as K. and G. are concerned is to make themselves into working farm hands."[41]

Becoming a farmer did not mean giving up the struggle for justice. Like Phoenix Settlement, Tolstoy Farm was far enough from the city to provide peace and natural beauty, but close enough for Gandhi and his fellow *satyagrahis* to remain active in the ongoing struggle. "This is a very important venture," Gandhi wrote of Tolstoy Farm. "Its roots go deep." Without the efforts of the entire community, those roots would lack supportive soil. "It is up to the *satyagrahis* who settle there," he wrote, "to make it bear sweet fruit by the way they live."[42]

Gandhi strove to make Tolstoy Farm self-sustaining, but the demands of the larger struggle forced him to rely upon outside supporters. In July 1910, for example, he received a case of bananas, pineapples, and Asian pears. Like contemporary advocates of local food, he would have preferred to grow all of his fruit on Tolstoy Farm. But in the midst of a larger struggle, he welcomed gifts of food. Farming was its own reward, but the social power of growing food—and sharing it—inspired Gandhi's love for farming. "Agriculture is the only real prayer and service," he declared in December 1914, some five months after leaving South Africa. After returning to India, he would continue to connect prayer, service, and agriculture by making farming a vital part of his social vision and his day-to-day life. Gandhi believed that the highest form of connection to

God was the struggle for justice. That struggle drove his dietary integrity and convinced him that farming could be a way to build a better world.[43]

THE ASHRAM AND THE WORLD

In 1915, soon after returning to India from South Africa, Gandhi embarked on a train journey across his native land. In the midst of the First World War, the Raj buzzed with energy. The war would shatter the Victorian world in which Gandhi had come of age. The great cities of the Raj had already swelled with people and modern technology. The rural landscape had also been transfigured. British canals had reshaped Indian agriculture, facilitating the consolidation of large landholdings, particularly in the breadbasket of the Raj, the Punjab. For British imperialists, the "improvement" of the land was connected to the "improvement" of nations. Agriculture had become a large-scale, technologically driven enterprise—like imperialism itself—pursued in the name of human advancement but maximizing profit for those at the top of an increasingly unequal society.[44]

Not all colonial officials endorsed an imperial approach to agriculture. One of India's most prominent scientists rejected the trend toward big farms. That scientist was none other than Robert McCarrison, the same doctor who lectured Gandhi on the need for meat and corrected the mahatma's views on vitamin D. During his tenure as the head of nutritional research in India, McCarrison became an ardent supporter of fresh, unprocessed food, and an early proponent of what would later be called organic agriculture. He and Gandhi differed on so many food-related issues that it must have been refreshing for them to find common ground.

McCarrison sent Gandhi several books on food, and agreed to be one of the few non-Indian members of the advisory board of the All-India Village Industries Association, an organization Gandhi founded in 1934 to advance his vision of sustainable rural development. Gandhi's emphasis on the interconnectedness of sustainable living found justification in the research that McCarrison conducted at the Nutrition Research Laboratories in the South Indian hill station of Coonoor. That research focused on the relationship between soil, food, and nutrition. The better the soil, McCarrison hypothesized, the more nutritious the crops. He saw such ecological links as part of what he called the Wheel of Life, and became an outspoken critic of pesticides and synthetic fertilizers. He also pioneered the connection between nutrition and health by studying the Hunza people, a rural community on India's northwest border. The Hunza ate an almost purely vegetarian diet with an emphasis on fruits, vegetables, whole grains, and dairy. McCarrison's research pushed doctors to reconsider the benefits of such a diet.[45]

McCarrison's views on agriculture were not entirely divorced from the discourses of his day. His research was part of a larger effort to measure the nutritional deficiencies of Indians and to suggest remedies. The colonial "discovery" of malnutrition proved to be yet another way for the British to justify their rule. Who else would help the poor Indians to feed themselves? To be sure, the British did not invent the problem of malnutrition. Hunger was all too real in colonial India. The regular famines decimating British India were only the most dramatic episodes in an unrelenting hunger that haunted India's poor. Scientists like McCarrison helped to quantify that hunger, but avoided linking it to the political and economic foundations of colonial inequality. Instead, colonial officials promoted a diet heavy with meat, dairy, and wheat and denigrated those Indians who preferred rice and *dal*. The colonial state anticipated the contemporary food empires that sell processed food throughout the world. Gandhi would be aghast at the power of what environmentalist Wenonah Hauter calls the foodopoly, "a small cabal of companies" that "control every aspect of our food system."[46]

It was an especially perfidious form of agricultural colonialism that Gandhi encountered in Champaran in 1917. Gandhi had been invited to that rural area of northeast India by a local farmer in order to investigate the suffering of farmers forced to grow indigo for wealthy European landowners. Indigo had once been a profitable crop, but its value had declined dramatically after artificial dyes flooded the market. Still, the landowners forced their sharecropping tenants to reserve a portion of their fields for the plant. Gandhi had scarcely arrived in Champaran when he was ordered to leave by a local official. He refused and was brought to court. With a boisterous crowd of farmers in attendance, the local judge wisely decided to set the prisoner free. After Gandhi and his colleagues interviewed some eight thousand farmers and catalogued their suffering, the central government passed legislation that ended the worst abuses of the system. Gandhi recognized that vast inequalities continued to mark the Indian countryside. During a visit to a small village scarred by poverty, he declared, "We can get *swaraj* only when we improve the lot of these people!"[47]

Improving the lot of the people meant improving their access to land. As a young man, Gandhi had lauded India's fecundity. In one of his earliest published articles, written in 1891, he proclaimed, "The soil of India is so rich that it can produce any vegetable you like." Over the years, he learned that many areas of India require extensive work to make them bear fruit. The biggest problem facing farmers was unequal access to fertile ground. At times, Gandhi seemed to endorse the redistribution of farmland. In 1927, he wrote privately that "agriculture is an industry which can only be improved when it receives state assistance." He envisioned "state assistance" as much more than subsidies. "In an ill-governed country," he explained, "I think with Thoreau that the citizen who resists the evil government must ignore property rights." Making clear that he was referring to agriculture, he added, "And without assurance of settled ownership, it is impossible to do much in the way of agriculture. I do not want to elaborate this thing. I have said sufficient to enable you to fill in the rest."[48]

Gandhi's reticence may have resulted from his desire to maintain the support of powerful Indian landlords and wealthy farmers. Rather than publicly endorse land redistribution, Gandhi championed cooperation between landlords (*zamindars*) and the peasants (*ryots*) who worked their land. He explained his vision in terms of what he called "trusteeship." It was "the duty of the ruler to be the trustee and friend of the people," but "the poor man must know that to a great extent poverty is due to his own faults and shortcomings." Such a patronizing defense of the status quo earned him the ire of activists like the Indian communist Rajani Palme Dutt, who spoke for many when he labeled Gandhi "the mascot of the bourgeoisie." Gandhi's defenders pointed to the fact that the mahatma expected a "model *zamindar*" to "reduce himself to poverty in order that the *ryot* may have the necessaries of life." But what if they refused? Gandhi's idea of wealth as trusteeship depended on individual *zamindars* voluntarily giving their wealth to the poor.[49]

Such voluntary redistribution was at the heart of one of the boldest social movements in independent India, a movement inspired by Gandhi and led by one of his most prominent disciples, Vinoba Bhave. How can you get land from large landowners to those who need it? Bhave's approach was radically simple; he asked nicely. Bhave walked from village to village asking large landholders to give one-sixth of their land to the poor. His campaign, the Bhoodan or "land-gift" movement, only partially succeeded. Some of the land that was gifted proved unsuitable for agriculture, and much of it was tied up in legal suits. In the words of historian Ramachandra Guha, "The Bhoodan movement must be reckoned a failure, but a spectacular one." While he did not end rural poverty, Bhave helped thousands of people to gain land while drawing attention to inequality.[50]

Despite his theory of trusteeship, Gandhi envisioned an egalitarian society. He wanted every village to be its own republic with "full powers," and imagined a "structure composed of innumerable villages" arranged in "ever-widening, never-ascending circles." As his emphasis on "never-ascending" makes clear, Gandhi's vision was horizontal rather than hierarchical. "Life will not be a pyramid with the apex sustained by the bottom," he declared. "It will be an oceanic circle whose centre will be the individual always ready to perish for the village." His oceanic circle was an antihierarchical utopia. Could such a utopia be realized even on a small scale?[51]

Before beginning the Salt March in the spring of 1930, Gandhi declared that he would not return to his ashram until India had gained independence. After eight months in prison, he emerged to an India still under British rule. He needed a new ashram. Increasingly focused on rural development, he wanted a place in India's countryside—the more remote, the better. Jamnalal Bajaj, one of his wealthiest supporters, owned land in Wardha, in the geographic center of India. With Bajaj's support, Gandhi would build his new ashram near a small village on Wardha's outskirts, a village that would be renamed Sevagram or "service village."

Early descriptions of Sevagram portray a bleak landscape of dust and heat. "From a distance," one ashram resident remembered, "Sevagram Ashram looked like a stockade in the middle of nowhere. . . . The land was flat and arid, baked dry much of the year by the burning sun." One of Gandhi's first initiatives was to plant trees. Eighty years later, the ashram is now a small arboretum, shaded by giant *peepal* trees, also known as banyan fig or *bodhi* trees. Although a species of fig, the *bodhi* tree's earthly fruits have never been as important as its spiritual produce. Its scientific name is fitting: *Ficus religiosa*. The Buddha is said to have attained enlightenment under a *bodhi* tree, and Gandhi sat under one during his daily prayers. Twice a day, a small group of ashram members and visitors continue to sit together under that tree to pray. They use the same prayers that Gandhi cherished, a combination of readings and songs from many of the world's faith traditions.[52]

When Gandhi came to Sevagram in the fall of 1933, his primary goal was, in his words, the "moral and physical advancement of the villages" of India. He wanted his ashram to be a model for local people, for all of India, and for the world. It would not be easy to make Sevagram live up to such high expectations. Part of the problem was the idealized image of rural life that Gandhi brought with him to Sevagram. Although he recognized many of the problems facing rural people, his utopian conception of village life justified his limited approach to agricultural inequality. Ultimately, however, it was the sheer scale of the problem that prevented any quick solutions. Gandhi knew that he could not end rural poverty without also abolishing British rule, untouchability, patriarchy, religious intolerance, and several other massive obstacles to India's freedom. He recognized the fundamental unity of the struggle for justice. While that unity fueled his desire to create a model community in Sevagram, it also pulled him away, both mentally and physically.[53]

On August 25, 1946, Gandhi left his ashram, bound for Delhi. From the train, he wrote an old friend and colleague that he hoped to be back in Sevagram in a week. He would never return. The seventeen months between his departure and his death in January 1948 contain many of the most dramatic events in his life and in the history of India. The British Raj would fall. The subcontinent would be torn in two. Independent India would go to war with its new neighbor, Pakistan. Millions of people would be killed or forced to flee their homes in a wave of violence that Gandhi fought against until the moment he was assassinated.

After leaving Sevagram and spending a few months in Delhi, Gandhi traveled to the remote region of Noakhali, near the northeast corner of India, where violence had erupted between Hindus and Muslims. There, he walked barefoot from village to village, cultivating peace one community at a time. His greatest success of this period, and perhaps the greatest success of his life, came not far from Noakhali in the great metropolis of Calcutta. In such a vast city, Gandhi could not combat violence by talking to individual people. He needed a way to communicate on a much vaster scale. As India and Pakistan emerged into a bloody freedom, Gandhi fought for peace with the only weapon he had left, a weapon he had perfected throughout his life. He fasted.

CHAPTER 7

Fasting

I will give you a talisman. Whenever you are in doubt, or when the self becomes too much with you, apply the following test. Recall the face of the poorest and the weakest man whom you may have seen, and ask yourself if the step you contemplate is going to be of any use to him. Will he gain anything by it? Will it restore him to a control over his own life and destiny? In other words, will it lead to *swaraj* for the hungry and spiritually starving millions? Then you will find your doubts and yourself melting away.

GANDHI, 1947

ON AUGUST 31, 1947, TWO WEEKS AFTER INDIA GAINED INDEPEN-
dence, Gandhi announced that he would fast unto death. Only one thing could save his life. The violence sweeping through the city of Calcutta would have to stop. Hindu versus Muslim, neighbor against neighbor—carnage had descended on the former capital of British India. In 1946, more than four thousand people had died when religious riots struck Calcutta. In 1947, by contrast, hundreds of thousands of lives, perhaps more than a million, would be lost in the bloodshed that followed independence. Gandhi bet his life against a wave of violence without precedent in the history of India.

The British were leaving. Their legacy included tea, cricket, and a land riven by nearly two hundred years of colonial rule. In their haste to depart, they left a range of unresolved questions, many stemming from the fact that not one, but two countries had gained freedom. As the British Raj split into a mostly Muslim Pakistan and a mostly Hindu India, millions of refugees streamed across the still-fresh borders. In Calcutta, Hindus fleeing East Pakistan (later Bangladesh) arrived with tales of atrocities and a commitment to vengeance. Armed gangs roamed the city. It seemed as if nothing could halt the bloodshed. Then Gandhi fasted.

Gandhi loved to fast. His most potent political weapon, the fast was also a crucial part of his diet. Relinquishing food from time to time was, he believed, a vital element of any healthy lifestyle. He carefully tracked the physical impact of his fasts, but going without food was never a purely physical process. Regardless of whether he was moved by politics or health, fasting was ultimately a form of prayer.

Fasting for religious reasons has a long and storied history; all of the world's major religions regard it as a key spiritual practice. The spiritual dimensions of fasting inspired Tolstoy to call it "an indispensable condition of a good life." Gandhi would have agreed. His diet was a way to break through the limitations of the ego, and fasting was his most powerful tool. For him, the role of fasting within Hinduism and Jainism was especially important. Many Hindus and Jains fast during festivals, on holy days, and as a personal act of spiritual growth.[1]

Fasting as a form of self-transcendence requires extraordinary discipline and can become a form of self-obsession. In the words of historian Sidney Mintz, "People who fast for some larger good are moved by a moral desire; they *will* against their own hunger." Willing against hunger in order to master the self can slide into obsessive self-destruction. Gandhi desired to transcend desire. His fasts reveal the power and the danger of that ancient spiritual quest.[2]

In the summer of 1947, as India gained its independence, Gandhi fasted to save Calcutta and penned his famous talisman. "Recall the face of the poorest and the weakest man whom you may have seen," he wrote, "and ask yourself if the step you contemplate is going to be of any use to him." Gandhi's fasts aimed to empower "the poorest and the weakest," and to bring swaraj to "the hungry and spiritually starving millions." By forgoing food, Gandhi challenged the British Empire and strove to heal a divided city. But he could not conquer his own desires. Like rejecting salt and sugar or limiting himself to only five foods per day, fasting was an effort at self-control through self-denial. Nothing testifies to his love for food, or the complicated ways he manifested that love, like Gandhi's hunger.[3]

"I eat like a bull," Gandhi declared in 1911. Later in life, he became famous for living with less—less money, less clothing, and less food. That austerity did not come easily. Many believe falsely, in the words of a close colleague, that the mahatma "was born so holy that he had a natural bent for fasting." "In reality," his friend remembered, he "was one of the hungriest men I have ever known." Gandhi struggled to let go of his attachment to food. He had to learn how to fast.[4]

Gandhi saw fasting as a form of natural healing. In 1925, he described the healing power of fasting with a characteristic blend of confidence, modesty, and humor. "With apologies to medical friends, but out of the fullness of my own experience and that of fellow-cranks," he declared, "I say without hesitation, fast (1) if you are constipated, (2) if you are anemic, (3) if you are feverish, (4) if you have indigestion, (5) if you have a headache, (6) if you are rheumatic, (7) if you are gouty, (8) if you are fretting and fuming, (9) if you are depressed, (10) if you are overjoyed; and you will avoid medical prescriptions and patent medicines." Juxtaposing physical ailments—constipation, anemia, fever—with psychological maladies like depression, Gandhi made evident his belief that fasting could heal both mind and body. At his most exuberant, he would claim that fasting could control plague, cholera, and dysentery. With time, he outgrew such farfetched claims. But he maintained his belief that fasts had healing power.[5]

Gandhi's personal experience confirmed the power of fasting, but left unclear why avoiding food could be so beneficial. One theory involved cleansing. "During fasting the body gets rid of many of its impurities," Gandhi declared. The human body does have the ability to "detox" or to cleanse itself of waste; such purification is the main job of the liver and the kidneys. Little evidence exists, however, to indicate that fasting aids the body's natural ability to cleanse itself of impurities.[6]

Despite his zeal, Gandhi stressed that fasting must be done carefully. "I know many cases," he wrote, "in which people who fasted have done themselves harm." One must not, he warned, alternate between feast and famine. In 1918, he ended a fast too abruptly and suffered indigestion as a result. Not only did he consume too much too quickly; he also ate a coriander rice dish, *ghens*, that is often prepared spicy. "If I had taken vegetable soup only," he wrote, "the painful result would certainly not have followed." He usually ended his fasts with a few sips of orange juice. A few hours later, he would add a small amount of fruit and a bit more juice. He often waited over a week before returning to his normal diet. One postfast diet entailed "only four tomatoes boiled with the skin off and a pineapple with a few monkey-nuts," as well as "a spoonful of the pawpaw vegetable and a lemon squash."[7]

Fasting did not eliminate the need for moderation. "A fast is not a substitute for eating less," he wrote. "The right way of ensuring that you eat less is that at every meal, you should ask them to serve you only once, and that too, only in a small quantity." Gandhi offered that advice from Yeravda prison, where such moderation might have come easily. A more challenging environment was the typical dinner party. "Unless we press the invited guest to overeat, we are considered to be extremely stingy," Gandhi complained. "On every holiday, we feel bound to prepare special dishes. On Sundays, we seem to think that we have the right to eat till we are sick." Regardless of the setting, so long as food was abundant the solution was clear: "Stop eating as soon as you feel that you have eaten so much as would permit you to eat the same quantity again." Fasts helped Gandhi eat less by breaking the connection between food and comfort. He cited an Italian proverb that declared, "He who eats more eats less," and explained in parentheses, "(because he shortens his days by gluttony)." He also quoted Seneca's dictum: *"Multos morbos multa fercula fuerunt"*—or, in Gandhi's rendering of the Latin, "Many dishes many diseases."[8]

Drinking water helped Gandhi go longer without food. "Drink as much cold water as you can," he advised those fasting. Dehydration is often mistaken for hunger. Unfortunately, fasting triggered in Gandhi a "distaste for water." He struggled with nausea during his fasts, and water made it worse. Lemon juice prevented the nausea, but Gandhi worried that lemon juice should not be permitted during fasting. He wrote doctors asking for advice, and eventually found that salt and carbonation made water more bearable.[9]

Gandhi's aversion to water forced him to grapple with the unpredictable nature of the fasting body. Even as he pushed the limits of physical and mental activity, he carefully monitored his health. "For three days and a half during the last fast," he wrote, "I worked practically from 4 o'clock in the morning till 8 o'clock in the evening." On the fourth day, however, he "developed a violent headache." Listening to his body and respecting his pain, he stopped all work and rested. "The following day I felt recuperated," he reported. "The feeling of exhaustion was gone, headache had almost subsided." On the sixth day, he felt "fresher still." On day seven, he reported, "I felt so fresh and strong that I was able to write with a steady hand my article on the fast." He was "in no hurry" to return to eating.[10]

Many fasting people find that their hunger pains vanish after the first few days. Part of the explanation for this involves the brain. The brain is only 2 percent of our body's mass, but it uses 20 percent of its energy. That energy normally comes in the form of glucose. After a few days of fasting, the body runs out of glucose, and the brain is forced to consume a backup fuel: ketone bodies, acidic compounds created from fatty acids. It takes the brain a few days to switch to ketones. During that time, the fasting brain struggles to operate with diminishing glucose stocks. When it finally gives up and begins to accept ketone bodies, the person fasting often experiences a sudden rush of well-being and clarity. Perhaps that cycle— from painful confusion to mysterious clarity—explains why so many mystics have embraced fasting as a method of spiritual transcendence.[11]

"Fasting is only good," Gandhi declared, "when it comes in answer to prayer and as a felt yearning of the soul." Where did he feel that yearning of the soul? In the pains of hunger or in their absence? His emphasis on overcoming desire might have led him to see fasting as a grueling test of willpower. Yet he encouraged those fasting to pamper their bodies as much as possible: to take a warm sponge bath daily, "sleep as much as possible in the open air," and "bathe in the morning sun." Rather than punishing the body, Gandhi saw fasting as a way to achieve peace in body, mind, and soul.[12]

He learned from his mother to associate fasting with spiritual growth. Rather than abstaining for a set period of time, she would break her fast on a particular day only if she saw the sun. A cloudy day meant no food. If the clouds suddenly parted, Gandhi would rush to proclaim the sun's emergence. If the clouds returned before his mother saw the light, she would shrug and explain that God did not want her to eat that day.

Gandhi learned from his mother that devotion can overcome the cravings of the body. Indeed, it was through such overcoming that he sought true devotion.[13]

Gandhi drew upon several faith traditions to explain his spiritual understanding of abstaining from food. He noted the "numerous fast days among Roman Catholics" and quoted the Bible in defense of the practice. When the mother of a Jewish friend became ill with a "severe attack of indigestion," Gandhi suggested "an extended Jewish fast." His own periods of abstinence often coincided with Hindu holy days, and he frequently cited passages from sacred Hindu texts that promoted fasting. His favorite example came from Islam. For Muslims, the holy month of Ramadan requires the devout to refrain from eating from sunrise to sundown. Gandhi lauded Muslims who observed Ramadan for "carrying out a self-imposed fast for full one month." He admired those who were "capable of undergoing such hardships not for the sake of any material or tangible gain, but for the sake of very intangible and purely spiritual benefit." After being jailed by the South African government, Gandhi championed the rights of Muslim prisoners to have special facilities for practicing the fast during Ramadan.[14]

Gandhi believed that fasting healed the rift between the body and the soul. After discussing the practice's physical benefits, he declared, "That is why our great men laid down for us certain religious observances like fasts, *rozas*, etc." The word *roza* refers to fasts undertaken by Muslims during Ramadan. Connecting Hindus and Muslims, Gandhi wrote, "The practice followed by many Hindus of eating only once a day during the *chaturmas* is based on considerations of health." During *chaturmas*, the four months of the monsoon, many Hindus undertake periodic fasts. Like Muslims, Gandhi argued, Hindus fasted for both religious reasons and for health; it was not necessary to choose between the two rationales. "Though almost all my fasts have been undertaken for a moral purpose," Gandhi explained, "being an inveterate diet reformer and a believer in fasting as a cure for many obstinate diseases, I have not failed to note their physical effects."[15]

Self-transcendence linked fasting's physical and spiritual dimensions. "No matter from what motive you are fasting," Gandhi told beginners, "during this precious time, think of your Maker, and of your relation to Him and His other creation." He strove to overcome the self by overcoming the craving for food, and encouraged everyone to "cease to think of food whilst you are fasting." While fasting might seem an odd time to try to transcend hunger, such transcendence was central to Gandhi's approach. "If the mind is hankering after food," he asked, "does it do any good to repress the desire and fast?" By letting go of his cravings, Gandhi strove to make his fasts a time of peace rather than conflict, a time of fulfillment rather than denial.[16]

Letting go of hunger requires discipline. Gandhi praised Muslims who saw in fasting "a discipline of the mind as well as of the body." He similarly stressed the importance of discipline when he lauded a Hindu relative for observing the Janmashtami fast, an annual celebration of Krishna. The mental concentration required to forgo food rendered fasting a spiritual discipline—but self-discipline need not be understood as self-denial. Gandhi believed fasting provided a period of physical, mental, and spiritual rest; he deemed such rest a form of grace. "There is only one simple way of winning divine grace," he wrote: "concentrating on one attachment or devotion to the exclusion of all others." During a successful fast, devotion to God eclipsed attachment to food.[17]

Prayer as purification was the key to success. "There is nothing as purifying as a fast, but fasting without prayer is barren," Gandhi wrote. "It is only a prayerful fast undertaken by way of penance to produce some effect on oneself which can be called a religious fast." His focus on self-purification was not a rejection of the world; instead, it entailed redirecting attention to the struggle against injustice. The opposite of purity is corruption. Gandhi understood the corruption of the soul and of the body as intimately related to the corruption of society. He borrowed from faith traditions to explain the social power of the self-discipline at the core of fasting. "Fasting," he wrote in a Christian idiom, should entail "crucifixion of the flesh with a corresponding freedom of the spirit." Like Jesus, he argued, we should fast in order to dedicate our lives to the greater good. Hindu texts reinforced Gandhi's belief in the power of fasting as a form of religious self-transformation. During one of his fasts in South Africa, Gandhi read a sacred verse every day. The final verse, saved for the twelfth day, praised the power of a fast to help the individual transcend the limits of the ego.[18]

The purifying power of the fast blended the spiritual, the physical, and the political—all in service of Gandhi's nonviolent approach to social change. "When people fast in a religious spirit and thus demonstrate their grief before God," he wrote, "hardest hearts are impressed." It was not just the "hardest hearts" of the British that were at stake. He also wanted to touch the hearts of those Indians who remained distant from the anticolonial struggle. "Fasting is regarded by all religions as a great discipline," he declared. "Those who voluntarily fast become gentle and purified by it." The simple act of relinquishing food was, therefore, a powerful tool. "A pure fast," he declared, "is a very powerful prayer." As a prayer, a fast transcends the distance between the self and the world; it "ennobles individuals and nations."[19]

Purity, discipline, perfection—the keywords that dominate Gandhi's writing on fasting echo the extreme austerity and the quest for perfection he brought to all facets of his diet. Like avoiding salt, sugar, and dairy, fasting promised self-transcendence through public service but risked devolving into an obsessive form of self-control. Consider Gandhi's emphasis on mastery and perfection. When it came to religious fasting, he proclaimed himself a "specialist par excellence." "I do not know any contemporary of mine who has reduced fasting and prayer to an exact science," he boasted, "and who has reaped a harvest so abundant as I have." Gandhi's extensive experience with fasting deserved a degree of self-congratulation. Nevertheless, his bragging reveals the urge for mastery that marked many facets of his diet, an urge complicated further by the political nature of many of his fasts. It matters that his self-designation as a "specialist par excellence" aimed to rally support for a grand experiment in political fasting.[20]

The year was 1919. The First World War had just ended. Thousands of Indians had fought and died for the British, and many hoped that the imperial government would reciprocate by granting India home rule. Instead, only a few moderate constitutional reforms were passed, and the British maintained the "emergency" suspension of civil liberties that had been enacted during the war. Feeling betrayed, Gandhi mobilized his supporters in opposition to British rule. He encouraged all Indians to stay home and dedicate themselves to fasting and "private religious devotion." What Gandhi framed as a day of fasting and prayer could also be described as a mass strike, known in India as a *hartal*. That is how the British saw it. A successful *hartal* threatened the foundations of the British Raj. If enough Indians withdrew their labor, the Raj would crumble.

Gandhi knew his protest was radical. By describing the protest as a day of fasting and prayer, he portrayed a radical protest as a religious act. In part, this was a clever publicity move. Gandhi aimed to win the support of moderates, both Indian and British, who might be more inclined to support religious meditation than a mass strike. His emphasis on the spiritual was, however, much more than a publicity stunt; he sincerely wanted the *hartal* to be grounded by prayer and fasting.

As with his opposition to salt and sugar, Gandhi argued that Indians had to achieve independence from bodily craving if they were to achieve independence from foreign rule. "I hope that both men and women," he wrote, "will observe the fast and devote the day to religious contemplation and try to understand the true nature of *satyagraha*." The true nature of *satyagraha* was spiritual and physical, as well as political. Gandhi praised "the efficacy of fasting as an aid to national progress, to the development of national ideals and to the attainment of restraint over our passions such as hunger, etc." National progress and personal progress were linked in this effort. Just as forgoing food helped the individual to eliminate harmful desires and physical impurities, so a political fast could empower Indians to rid their body politic of the scourge of imperialism.[21]

What if the desire for dominance and mastery that Gandhi brought to his own body was reproduced on a national scale? The mahatma saw political fasting as the essence of nonviolent *satyagraha*, but he also worried that fasting could become a form of coercion that was the opposite of nonviolent. Hunger strikes were often used to pressure the opposition, but such coercion struck him as a form of violence. From his early struggles with vegetarianism to his opposition to chocolate, he used his diet to deepen his practice of nonviolence. Fasting was the pinnacle of his dietary *ahimsa*—but also its greatest test. To be fully nonviolent, Gandhi believed, a fast could not become coercive. How could he use fasts to change the world without forcing others to change?

THE LOVER AND THE TYRANT

Fasting as a form of protest has a long history in India, but Gandhi learned to see fasting as a political tool in England. Among his teachers were British women who fasted for the right to vote. In London in 1909, Gandhi attended a suffragette meeting at St. James's Hall. Afterward, he penned a glowing report of the suffragettes' use of the hunger strike. Arrested and unjustly treated as "second class" prisoners, several suffragettes had refused food. "One of them ate nothing for six days," Gandhi reported, "some others for five days." He admired the activists for their discipline and their determination. Like them, he would employ the fast as a way to attack injustice within and beyond jail. Could he do so without turning hunger into a weapon of coercion? That challenge was especially tricky when the conflict he aimed to resolve occurred within his own family.[22]

In July 1913, Gandhi learned that his son, Manilal, had been having an affair with Jeki Mehta, the daughter of one of his closest supporters. Gandhi fasted for a week, and then vowed to eat only one meal a day for the next year. His fast was meant to atone for his own failure as a father and as the leader of the ashram in which both Manilal and Jeki lived. His actions also had a direct impact on the couple. Manilal vowed to remain celibate for several years and to postpone any plans to marry. Jeki cut short her long hair and took to wearing white, the traditional color of widows. Gandhi's decision to fast over such a personal matter is complicated by the fact that a few days before learning of the affair, he had considered fasting in response to a very different calamity. Thousands of white miners had gone on strike near Johannesburg; the authorities had responded with violence, and a dozen miners had been killed. Gandhi was deeply troubled by the violence and suggested to a close friend that they should respond by having only one meal a day for a year—precisely the formula he would use a few days later. His friend had talked him out of the partial fast, but the idea remained, ready to be implemented in matters we might see as more personal than political, but that Gandhi saw as both.[23]

Gandhi had for years experimented with eating only one meal per day. The practice served as a bridge between his body, his family, and the political change he hoped to create in South Africa. Right after completing his "penance" in response to the affair between Manilal and Jeki, Gandhi found yet another reason to undertake his "one meal" regimen: a mass strike of Indian laborers. Gandhi led a march of striking workers and was arrested. From jail, he pledged to "live on one meal a day" until the strike was victorious. A month later, after the police fired on some of the striking miners, he again proclaimed that he would restrict himself to one meal a day as a sign of "inward mourning." What does it say about the politics of Gandhi's hunger that he turned to meal restriction for multiple causes simultaneously? Over thirty years later, in 1945, he himself admitted, "In South Africa, I used to fast on any pretext. I must have taken only one meal a day for more than a year." We might praise such fasting for linking Gandhi's body to multiple causes—from the integrity of his family and his ashram to the struggle of the Indian community in South Africa. Yet there is something self-centered about Gandhi's repeated insertion of his own body into these disparate spheres and causes. By positioning his hunger at the center of these struggles, did Gandhi demonstrate the social power of self-transcendence or the hidden egotism of self-suffering? In any case, it seems disingenuous to publicly frame as a sacrifice a dietary practice he had long embraced as a form of healthful living.[24]

After the strike ended, Gandhi continued the practice of eating only one meal a day—now for reasons of health. He would engage in such dietary restrictions from time to time throughout the rest of his life. Meanwhile, he would repeatedly lament the fact that the poor in India had to live on "one meal per day." He saw no contradiction in choosing to eat only one meal while denouncing the deprivation forced on India's poor. Fasting was a way to relate to those who went without food by necessity rather than by choice. For many poor Indian villagers, Gandhi stated, "life is a process of slow starvation." "In Bihar," he told one audience, "the majority of people subsist on a stuff called *sattu* which is useless as nourishment." *Sattu*, or maize flour, was not as useless as Gandhi believed, but it was insufficient for a healthy diet. "When I saw people swallowing this *sattu*," he told one audience, "my eyes used to blaze with fire. If you were to have such food to eat, how long would you survive?" To a group of wealthy merchants, he declared bluntly, "People are dying of starvation." Speaking of India's poorest citizens, he told another audience, "It is our duty to dress them first and then dress ourselves, to feed them first and then feed ourselves."[25]

Forgoing food did not by itself mean less hunger for the poor. Gandhi recognized that merely eating less was not sufficient to help those starving. Similarly, wearing fewer clothes did not mean there would be more clothing for others. He used his fasts, like his simple loincloth, as a way to "be in touch with the life of the poorest of the poor." Being in touch with the poor, though, was not enough. Fasting in solidarity with the starving meant little unless coupled with a plan to end the inequalities that created mass hunger.[26]

Gandhi recognized that his fasts were made by choice, and were thus totally different from the chronic starvation of the poor, what he called "an eternal compulsory fast." But his fasts were not unrelated to the tragedy of mass starvation. By using fasts to heal his body, Gandhi hoped to have more energy to work toward a world where no one suffered from lack of food. In 1944, he encouraged his colleagues to end the "starvation of millions" in Bengal and elsewhere. "The claims of the famishing millions" should be "the first charge on their care and attention."[27]

Gandhi decried the inequality that drove mass hunger in India, but never used a fast to directly attack that inequality. Was fasting against corrupt landlords or the uneven distribution of land too coercive for the mahatma? The closest he came to fasting against economic inequality was in the spring of 1918, when he fasted in order to resolve a strike involving the millworkers of Ahmedabad, a large industrial city in his home state of Gujarat. Gandhi's involvement in that strike was one of his first political acts after returning to India from South Africa—and one that blurred the lines between fasting as self-purification and as coercion. A leaflet most likely written in part by Gandhi declared that the fast was "not intended to influence the employers." Rather, the goal was to rally the workers themselves to remain on strike. Refusing work created tremendous hardship for the millworkers, some of whom challenged Gandhi that it was easy for him to endorse the strike given that he was not suffering deprivation. It was all too easy, Gandhi admitted, for those who had "plenty of food" to "advise staunchness even unto death." Challenged by the millworkers, Gandhi promised that he would fast until a reasonable settlement had been reached.[28]

Gandhi understood his fast as an expression of religious devotion. "It was a sacred moment for me," he explained. "My faith was on the anvil." In the midst of the struggle, a Christian friend sent Gandhi a telegram with a sentence from the Bible: "Greater love has no man than this, that he lay down his life for his friends." Gandhi praised the telegram as "the most touching and the truest of all" the correspondence he received regarding the fast. He shared the line with his son Devdas, and explained that it communicated "the significance of the fast very clearly." "The peace which I knew at the time of that fast was," Gandhi declared, "no mere human experience."[29]

The impact of the fast on the millworkers was, according to Gandhi, "electrifying." He claimed that they "awoke to the reality of their soul, a new consciousness stirred in them and they got strength to stand by their pledge." He wrote his Christian friend that "the existence of God was realized by the mass of men before me as soon as the fast was declared." Gandhi might have overstated the significance of his fast to the workers; his description of their awakening reeks of self-importance. Yet the strikers had good reason to hope that Gandhi's fast would resolve the conflict. The leader of the mill owners, Ambalal Sarabhai, was Gandhi's personal friend. "A gentlemen in every sense of the term," in Gandhi's words, Sarabhai had become one of the mahatma's most important supporters. Their relationship was a source of hope for the workers, but for Gandhi it produced an ethical dilemma. How could he ensure that his fast was directed only at supporting the strikers and not at coercing Sarabhai and the other mill owners?[30]

In the midst of the struggle, Gandhi sent a letter to Sarabhai. "Be guided by your sense of justice," he urged his friend, "rather than your desire to see that I break my fast." The next day, a settlement was reached. Unfortunately, the mahatma told residents of his ashram, the settlement was "quite unacceptable." "Deny it as emphatically as I may, the people cannot but feel that the mill-owners have acted under pressure of my fast," he explained. "My weak condition left the mill-owners no freedom." Given that the means must match the ends, Gandhi did not want to champion freedom by denying it to his adversaries. How could he fight against injustice without pressuring others to change?[31]

The question of coercion arose even more profoundly during the noncooperation movement. After Gandhi asked all Indians to give up British goods and to retreat from supporting the Raj, one correspondent asked, "Would it be regarded as coercion on my relatives if I made them give up tea by resorting to fasting?" Gandhi replied that fasting to make one's family give up tea was indeed coercion. If one wanted to change the habits of a family member, one should "reason with them patiently." "Resorting to fasting simply because others do not stop doing a particular thing is a form of blackmail," he declared, "and that is coercion."[32]

In his own life, however, Gandhi often turned to fasts to reform the habits of others. Recall his recourse to a nut-free "partial starvation" in response to his wife's belief in untouchability, or his fast in response to his son's affair with Jeki Mehta. Or consider three entries in Gandhi's diary for 1915. On June 1, he wrote, "Noticed falsehood among the boys. And so started a fast. Lying admitted. Broke the fast in the evening." On July 17, he wrote, "Ba washed Deva's dhoti. Seen doing so. Told a lie. Could not control my anger. Went at her. Vowed to fast for 14 days if she should wash anything of Deva's, even a handkerchief. May God help." On September 11, he wrote, "Started a fast because Vrajlal had smoked." Gandhi fasted against lying, untouchability, and smoking. He also fasted to change his children, his students, and his wife. His opposition to coercion was not always evident.[33]

Despite his own behavior at home, Gandhi recoiled at the prospect of fasts roiling families and communities across India. He was troubled by the zealous methods of his most ardent supporters. When some Indian parents refused to withdraw their children from a government school, activists inspired by what they took to be Gandhian tactics "fasted until the poor bewildered parents had complied with their request." Gandhi lectured the activists that such pressure "bordered on violence, for we had no right to make people conform to our opinion by fasting." He distinguished between fasting "for enforcing one's right" and fasting "for imposing one's opinion on another." That distinction proved difficult to apply in practice.[34]

When a volunteer fasted in order to goad others toward noncooperation, Gandhi responded by clarifying the proper role of a fast. "Whilst your action shows the purity of your heart and the spirit of sacrifice," he wrote, "it is hasty and possibly thoughtless." The tactic must be used carefully. "Fasting for the purpose of showing one's displeasure or disappointment can hardly be justified," he explained. The foundation of a fast "must be penance or purification." The method must never become a form of "pressure." "We must give to everyone," Gandhi concluded, "the same freedom of action and speech that we claim for ourselves."[35]

If Gandhi did not want his followers to fast against fellow Indians, he also rejected the idea that noncooperation fasting was directed against the government. He declared, "The coming fast is thus in no way to be interpreted as designed to put pressure upon the Government." According to Gandhi, the action's primary purpose was to purify and strengthen those who had already decided to noncooperate. Gandhi never linked the noncooperation fasting to any particular demands, as he would other fasts. Yet to suggest that the campaign worked only by influencing those who were fasting would be to fundamentally undersell the power of Gandhi's method. He himself suggested that fasts often work by influencing others. To avoid the risk of coercion, he introduced a dichotomy that encapsulates many of the ambiguities and contradictions of Gandhi's views. He claimed that fasts work best when the intended audience consists of "a lover" and not "a tyrant."[36]

"You cannot fast against a tyrant," Gandhi declared, "for it will be as a piece of violence done to him." Only a relationship based on love could allow a fast to be a source of positive change rather than negative violence. "Fasting can only be resorted to against a lover," he made clear, "not to exhort rights but to reform him, as when a son fasts for a father who drinks." It is striking that Gandhi chose to imagine a son using hunger to influence a father, rather than the situation that was much more common in his own life—the father fasting to reform the son. Perhaps he recognized that his use of fasts as a means of influencing his family would strike most audiences as patently coercive. For a more political example, Gandhi turned to the strike in Ahmedabad. He had fasted, he argued, "against 'lovers'—the mill-hands, and not against the owners—'the tyrants.'" The fact that he was on close terms with the owners complicates such a simple division. Was Ambalal Sarabhai, a man who Gandhi considered not only a patron but a friend, really a "tyrant" rather than a "lover"? Gandhi left unclear how to distinguish between the two, or between a nonviolent attempt at "reform" and a violent effort to coerce.[37]

Gandhi's distinction between the lover and the tyrant came in response to a protest against caste oppression in the South Indian town of Vaikom. For generations, the lowest castes had been denied access to Vaikom's temple. In the early 1920s, a protest movement aimed to open the temple's doors. One of the leaders of the protest suggested using a fast to convince the local maharaja. Gandhi opposed the idea of fasting against the maharaja, and introduced the lover-tyrant distinction to explain his opposition.[38]

We cannot understand that distinction, or Gandhi's response to the protest in Vaikom, without examining his relationship with caste. Like his views on race, his relationship with caste changed dramatically over the course of his life. Unlike the fierce antipathy he developed toward racial inequality, however, Gandhi never fully discarded his belief in some form of caste. He strongly opposed untouchability, but his opposition to caste more generally was constrained by his belief in a division of labor and his desire to maintain unity in the struggle against imperialism. He did not want to alienate powerful high-caste Hindus whose support he needed to fight the British. Despite such pressure, Gandhi publicly denounced untouchability and earned the ire of some orthodox Hindus by championing the rights of untouchables, now often referred to as *Dalits*, a word that means those who are oppressed or broken. Gandhi preferred the term *Harijan*, son of God. The word *Harijan* aimed to remove the curse of untouchability, but was seen as paternalistic by many low-caste activists. It did not help that Gandhi opposed untouchability but stopped short of attacking caste. He also rejected the use of nonviolent civil disobedience in the struggle against caste oppression. His limitations were made apparent in his most infamous fast.[39]

In 1933, the British announced that separate electorates were to be granted to Dalits. The most renowned Dalit leader, Dr. Bhimrao Ramji Ambedkar, championed the idea that Dalits should be able to elect their own representatives. Ambedkar recognized that Dalits needed political power if they were to fight for their rights. As an oppressed minority, they would never be able to gain power unless their votes were counted separately from those of the higher castes. Whether out of sincere concern for caste inequality or as a way to further divide Indians, the British agreed.[40]

Gandhi responded by beginning a fast unto death. He refused to eat until separate electorates were withdrawn. Recognizing that if Gandhi died it might lead to widespread violence against Dalits, Ambedkar reluctantly relinquished the idea of separate electorates. Gandhi framed his fast as an effort to oppose untouchability. For Ambedkar and many of his followers, the fast was a betrayal of the Dalit cause. To his credit, Gandhi poured energy into a public campaign against untouchability;

imprisoned again, he launched yet another fast when his jailers denied him the opportunity to work on the campaign. "Life ceases to interest me if I may not do Harijan work without let or hindrance," he wrote. On April 30, 1933, he sent a telegram to the Secretary of the Home Department. The telegram explained that "for reasons wholly unconnected with government and solely connected with Harijan Movement," Gandhi had to follow a "call from within" to undergo a twenty-one-day "unconditional irrevocable fast." He would allow himself only water, baking soda, and salt.[41]

By fasting, Gandhi coerced Ambedkar into giving up separate electorates. Ambedkar would remain a fierce critic of the mahatma. In 1945, he published a scathing critique entitled *What Congress and Gandhi Have Done to the Untouchables*. Ambedkar used Gandhi's own words to paint him as a procaste reactionary. He quoted Gandhi: "I believe that if Hindu Society has been able to stand it is because it is founded on the caste system." To demonstrate the mahatma's unwillingness to endorse intercaste marriage or intercaste dining, Ambedkar again quoted Gandhi: "I believe that interdining or intermarriage are not necessary for promoting national unity." For stronger evidence, Ambedkar might also have quoted Gandhi defending restrictions on "interdining" as an opportunity for the "cultivation of will-power and the conservation of certain social virtues." Instead, he shifted from an attack on Gandhi's blinkered views on caste to a more general critique of his approach to the world and to food in particular. He quoted a passage in which Gandhi defended his opposition to interdining by denouncing the very act of eating: "Taking food is as dirty an act as answering the call of nature. The only difference is that after answering call of nature we get peace while after eating food we get discomfort. Just as we perform the act of answering the call of nature in seclusion so also the act of taking food must also be done in seclusion."

Such revulsion at the act of eating shines a harsh light on Gandhi's fasts and chronic caloric restriction. What Gandhi portrayed as a spiritual quest for personal and social health instead emerges as an unhealthy rejection of food and the body. After quoting Gandhi's bizarre and disturbing comparison between eating and "answering the call of nature," Ambedkar concluded, "He has outdone the most orthodox of orthodox Hindus. It is not enough to say that it is an argument of a cave man. It is really an argument of a mad man."[42]

Ambedkar linked the extremity of Gandhi's diet to the limitations of his politics, but the portrait he presented was more static than the reality. Gandhi's views on food and eating changed dramatically over time, as did his views on caste. Early in life, he repeatedly advised different castes to eat separately, but toward the end of his life he made a point of eating with Dalits, and encouraged others to do so as well. In 1935, in an article entitled "Caste Has to Go," he wrote that there "should be no prohibition of intermarriage or interdining." In June 1940, a Brahmin widow asked if she should interdine with Harijans "or any other non-Brahmin caste." Gandhi encouraged her "to disregard the restriction on interdining and the like as a hindrance to spiritual and national progress." As with interdining, he reversed his opposition to intermarriage. For years, he publicly opposed intercaste marriages; later, he openly advocated for them. Gandhi became a mahatma by learning from his mistakes and changing his mind. His fasts, which he often framed as a form of personal penance, helped him to grow. And because he made them public, others learned as well.[43]

Despite Gandhi's public rejection of coercion, his fasts worked by applying pressure, often to those "lovers" who already cared deeply about him. His rejection of coercion might be seen as blatantly hypocritical, but his goal was self-transcendence through self-control. Only by disciplining himself did he believe he could truly educate and inspire others. Self-control, vital to many facets of his diet, was foundational to his fasts. As with the rejection of salt and sugar, fasting blurred the line between self-control and social control. What Gandhi saw as a personal struggle against his ego became a way for him to enforce his dietary goals on his family and his closest followers. Could such a tactic work on an entire city? Was it ethical to try?[44]

THE CALCUTTA MIRACLE

"Can you fast against the *goondas*?" Gandhi's friend and colleague, Chakravarti Rajagopalachari, known affectionately as Rajaji, chose his words carefully. It was September 1, 1947, and the mahatma had just announced that he would forgo food in order to end the violence in Calcutta. Rajaji urged him to reconsider. The Hindi word *goonda* perfectly captures the inveterate thugs (to use another word of Indian origin) that

Rajaji worried would remain untouched by the fast. Gandhi, however, refused to blame the violence on criminals. He redirected attention back to his own failings and those of others like him. "It is we who make *goondas*," he declared. "Without our sympathy and passive support, the *goondas* would have no legs to stand upon." It was the apathy of the good, he believed, that allowed the violence of the bad. His fast aimed "to touch the hearts of those who are behind the *goondas*." He fasted to inspire everyone, himself included, to confront the violence they abetted and to take concrete steps to bring peace. He bet his life that the common citizens of Calcutta could be convinced to take a stand for peace. Many lives hinged on this gamble. "Supposing you die," Rajaji argued, "the conflagration would be worse." The mahatma's death could trigger waves of violent retribution. "I shall have done my bit," Gandhi replied. "More is not given a man to do."[45]

In less than a year, Gandhi would give his life in the cause of Hindu-Muslim unity. He did not want to die, but by the time the assassin's bullets cut through his body, he had already placed himself on the sacrificial altar. He knew the risks he faced. The possibility of his death was vital to the success of his fast in Calcutta. Fasting transformed Gandhi's physical weakness into moral strength; as his body wasted away, his fragility touched the hearts of the people.

Even before he began to fast, Gandhi had used his bodily safety as a gambit for peace. He had moved into a Muslim house in an area torn by violence, and invited the leading Muslim political figure in Calcutta, Huseyn Shaheed Suhrawardy, to live with him as his guest. From the perspective of many of Calcutta's Hindus, it would have been hard to find a greater villain than Suhrawardy. Angry Hindus appeared in front of Gandhi's residence, threatening violence. Gandhi confronted the mob and managed to pacify their anger, but the calm would prove temporary. On August 31, a crowd converged on Gandhi's headquarters. They carried the body of a Hindu man who claimed to have been knifed by a Muslim. By evening of the next day, fifty people had been killed.[46]

Gandhi announced his fast. He hoped it might "touch the hearts of all the warring elements." He would return to eating only "if and when sanity returns to Calcutta." On the second day of the fast, a hopeful quiet fell upon the city. In a telling metaphor, Gandhi declared, "The leaven has begun to work." Like baking bread, fasting required patience. He did not expect "to be able to control all the *goondas* in the city." He understood the power of his fast as a direct result of his own spiritual progress, and regretted that he did not have "the requisite degree of purity, detachment and steadfastness of mind." Because he was not perfect, his fast could not be all-powerful. By revealing his imperfections, however, his fast helped him grow. When Rajaji asked why he had chosen to add lemon juice to his water, something he normally avoided, Gandhi responded that he had "allowed it out of weakness." In that small moment of humility, he demonstrated how fasting helped him recognize his own limitations and simultaneously transcend them.[47]

Gandhi's personal struggle inspired a social transformation that is justly known as the Calcutta miracle. Gangs brought him their weapons. The police undertook a twenty-four-hour sympathy fast. Throughout the city, people began to worry about Gandhi. It was if the future of all Calcutta hinged on one man's health. "People would begin to feel uncomfortable," one contemporary wrote, whenever news emerged of Gandhi's fragility. Preoccupied with the mahatma's well-being, "The grocer's boy, the rickshaw-puller, the office clerk, the school and college students would scan the news columns early in the morning and listen to the radio throughout the day and feel more and more personally involved in the situation."[48]

On September 4, Gandhi told a group of Hindu demonstrators to "go immediately among the Muslims and assure them full protection." He added, "If you do not now hurry up it may be too late. I cannot last for many more days." Later that evening, Gandhi welcomed a deputation of influential religious and political leaders. The group included the president and secretary of the Bengal Hindu Mahasabha, the editor of an influential Sikh daily, and a representative of the Muslim League. All came to plead for Gandhi's life. Collectively, they signed a document pledging their support for peace. "We the undersigned," the document declared, "promise Gandhiji that now that peace and quiet have been restored in Calcutta once again, we shall never allow communal strife in the city and shall strive unto death to prevent it."[49]

Even at the moment of triumph, Gandhi worried that people had acted out of coercion rather than personal conviction. "If a single step was taken under pressure of the fast, not from conviction," he declared, "it would cause oppression." What if the fast had coerced people into holding new convictions? Rather than admit that coercion had played some role in the success of the fast, Gandhi focused on the power of self-purification. "The function of my fast is to purify," he instructed the delegation, "to release our energies by overcoming our inertia and mental sluggishness, not to paralyse us or to render us inactive." Purifying the city did not mean arresting the *goondas*. True purification meant eliminating violence from the hearts and minds of every citizen of Calcutta. "My fast isolates the forces of evil," he continued. "The moment they are isolated they die, for evil by itself has no legs to stand upon."[50]

Having been convinced that the Calcutta miracle would last, Gandhi prepared to end his fast. "I have the will power to live and would like to live," he declared, "but I do not want to be deceived in order to live." He cautioned against complacency. If the violence was to end permanently, the people of Calcutta would have to work actively to maintain the peace. "I expect that the Hindus and Muslims here will not force me to undertake a fast again," he warned. Ultimately, he put his faith in God. "May God grant wisdom to everyone," he told the crowd that gathered to watch him end his fast. A group of girls began to sing one of his favorite songs: "*Ishwar Allah tere nam, sabko sanmati de Bhagwan* [Your name is Ishwar, Allah, you are the greatest God.]" "Above all, there is God, our witness," Gandhi declared and took a sip of orange juice.[51]

Mangoes and Mahatmas

R. came in this morning. He brought some luscious mangoes.
I fretted to find that you were not here to share them.

GANDHI, 1920

O N A WARM MAY MORNING IN THE SPRING OF 1920, GANDHI looked at a box of mangoes and yearned to share. His response to those "luscious mangoes" reveals his diet at its most human. His delight for the simple pleasures of the fruit merged with the joy of sharing. Twenty years later, another box of mangoes arrived as "medicine" for a group of patients he was helping to treat. The sweet aroma of the fruit led him to eat a few himself. It is unclear how many he devoured, but his response was ferocious. "Mango is a cursed fruit," he declared. "We must get used to not treating it with so much affection."[1]

In 1920, Gandhi delighted in mangoes; twenty years later, he cursed them. What accounts for this dramatic shift? As a young man, he radically changed his relationship to food: what was once a treat for his palate became sustenance for his soul. But that evolution occurred well before the earlier box of mangoes arrived. By 1920, he had rejected sweets, experimented with a saltless diet, and vowed to eat only five food items per day. Yet he remained eager to share those mangoes. The fact that the second batch arrived as medicine helps to explain his anguish at having eaten them. Yet Gandhi often rejected food even when it was not meant for others—vowing to treat ginger as "forbidden," for instance, and criticizing chocolate. Conversely, the possibility of sharing did not automatically lead him to delight in flavorful treats. On the contrary, he condemned the routine giving of sweets as a harmful habit that should be abolished.

The ambivalence in Gandhi's relationship to mangoes reveals a larger tension at the center of his diet, a tension between seeing food as an instrument of service and celebrating food for its own sake. The author E. B. White once wrote, "I arise in the morning torn between a desire to improve (or save) the world and a desire to enjoy (or savor) the world. This makes it hard to plan the day." Gandhi too struggled with that balance, as his mango travails make clear. At stake was his ability to live a life that was passionate but not selfish, joyful but not lustful. The difficulty of discerning healthy desire from unhealthy lust is revealed by the most important detail in Gandhi's encounter with the mangoes he yearned to share: their intended recipient.[2]

Sarala Devi Chaudhurani, a dynamic anticolonial activist, was the founder of one of India's oldest women's organizations. When Gandhi saw her for the first time, she was conducting an orchestra as it performed a piece she had written in honor of the Indian National Congress. In 1919, Gandhi met Chaudhurani in Lahore and reported "bathing in her deep affection." He was fifty. She was forty-seven. Both were married. Over the next year, the two exchanged a series of increasingly intimate letters. Their relationship became sufficiently close that Gandhi deemed it a "spiritual marriage." What that relationship entailed has galvanized rumor-mongers, but no evidence suggests a physical dimension. Nevertheless, their relationship was sufficiently improper that Gandhi's son asked him to end it.[3]

In December 1920, some seven months after Gandhi wrote Chaudhurani about those luscious mangoes, he sent her a detailed note explaining why their relationship could not continue as it was. "Spiritual partners can never be physically wedded," he explained. "Have we that exquisite purity, that perfect coincidence, that perfect merging, that identity of ideals, that self-forgetfulness, that fixity of purpose, that trustfulness? For me I can answer plainly that it is only an aspiration. I am unworthy to have that companionship with you." With deep regret, Gandhi concluded, "I am too physically attached to you to be worthy of enjoying that sacred association with you." He had tried to transcend the physical but, as with those "cursed" mangoes, he had failed.[4]

Gandhi strove to avoid temptations that pulled him away from his purpose and into the desires of the body, but his goal was not to transcend the body entirely. He could walk away from Sarala Devi Chaudhurani, reject chocolate, and perhaps even avoid mangoes, but completely escaping food was not his goal. He recognized the limitations of his embodied being, but also believed that his diet could empower his spiritual growth. The link between his food, his body, and his soul led him to declare, "A perfectly moral person alone can achieve perfect health." "The body is so closely bound to the soul," he explained, "that one whose body is pure will be pure in mind too." Gandhi's connection between morality and health inspired many of his greatest dietary achievements. His emphasis on perfection and purity speaks, however, to the Victorian obsessions that turned his relationship to food into a self-centered struggle to overcome the self—a struggle that was, by definition, self-defeating.[5]

It would be easy to dismiss Gandhi's efforts to control his body as the self-centered obsessions of a Victorian prude. But as the philosopher Aakash Singh Rathore has written, "The discovery of oneself requires inwardness, turning away (*pratyahara*)." The ultimate goal of Gandhi's inwardness was not control of his body; he wanted to change the world. As a young man in South Africa, he prepared a series of articles on diet and health in the midst of an epic confrontation with South Africa's racist government. In the fall of 1942, imprisoned by the British, he took the opportunity to author another text on diet. Although separated by more than three decades, these writings are remarkably similar. The basic principles of his diet remained constant throughout his adult life. Equally consistent was the fact that his dietary concerns would not wait for politics, even dramatic conflicts like his struggle against South African racism and his final battle against British imperialism. Gandhi's diet did not replace more political concerns. His diet *was* political.[6]

Gandhi's evolution from lawyer for the wealthy to advocate for the needy was intimately bound up with his diet. He opposed the salt tax while exploring how to cut salt from his diet. He championed the rights of Indian indentured laborers forced to harvest sugar in terrible conditions, and he rejected sugar itself. As his food came to reflect his purpose, he learned to eat better and to live better—to eat and to live in the service of others. At least, that was his goal. A cynic might conclude that the noble purpose-driven understanding Gandhi brought to his diet only drove him to become ever more obsessively self-focused. The truth is more complicated.

As his relationship with Sarala Devi Chaudhurani and those "cursed" mangoes makes clear, Gandhi's conflicted relationship to the body defied the distinction between self and society by linking gender, sexuality, and diet. He strove to empower women as leaders, and saw culinary reform (and particularly raw food) as a way to free women from labor in the kitchen. His embodied politics subverted the colonial practice of equating women with the body and men with the mind—although his aversion to bodily pleasure could also reinforce such a gendered divide. "In much of philosophy, religion, and literature," writes the political scientist Janet Flammang, "food is associated with body, animal, female, and appetite—things civilized men have sought to overcome with knowledge and reason." For Gandhi, appetite was decidedly male. He lumped together the desire for flavor and the desire for sex in ways that could position women as seductive objects to be avoided, like chocolate. Gandhi believed women were especially capable of overcoming desire; compared to men, he felt, they were more pure and thus more powerful. His praise of female purity was patronizing, and his patriarchal instincts led him to force many of his dietary practices on his wife and their children.[7]

Later in life, one of Gandhi's sons, Harilal, wrote him an angry letter. "Not to take salt, not to take ghee," the letter declared, "not to take milk has no bearing on character. You say this is necessary in pursuit of self-control. But my view is that even before one cultivates self-control, there are other even more desirable qualities that need to be stressed—such as being unselfish." Harilal had a point. By imposing his dietary preferences on his family, Gandhi indulged in selfishness. His diet became a form of control.[8]

Given that controlling his body at times overlapped with controlling his wife and children, Gandhi's obsession with diet might be criticized as a masculinist fixation. In our day, men who reduce their caloric intake are often praised for self-control, while women who make similar choices are labeled obsessive and potentially self-destructive. Gandhi himself defied the gender norms of his day; as political psychologist Ashis Nandy wrote, "It was colonial India, still preserving something of its androgynous cosmology and style, which ultimately produced a trans-cultural protest against the hyper-masculine world view of colonialism, in the form of Gandhi." The British routinely feminized Indians, especially Hindus, in an effort to protect and justify British rule. Gandhi managed to attack British colonialism without moving to the opposite extreme of defending some kind of hypermasculinity. His diet facilitated his efforts to challenge prevailing ideas of gender and sexuality. As postcolonial theorist Leela Gandhi has written, blending "anticolonialism, vegetarianism, and a formative antipathy to 'modern civilization,' Gandhian *ahimsa* or nonviolence is, indeed, predicated upon a rigorous refusal of heteronormative masculinity."[9]

Gandhi's rejection of certain norms of masculinity coincided with his rejection of sex and his efforts to "conquer" his palate. Was he replacing one form of control with another? In confronting the messiness of gender, sex, and food, he transgressed certain social lines while strengthening others. The note he sent Sarala Devi Chaudhurani concerning those "luscious mangoes" brims with longing and desire. After describing the newly arrived fruit, Gandhi yearned for Chaudhurani's presence and noted that he awoke "at our usual time but turned in again. I did not watch the sunrise. Had you been here I know you would have dragged me to watch His Majesty coming in." Pining to share a sunrise and a case of mangoes, Gandhi revealed the absence at the heart of desire, but also the way in which attending to absence can become a kind of presence. "To take pleasure in an activity is to engage in that activity while being absorbed in it," writes the philosopher Talbot Brewer. Elaborating an old Aristotelian conception of pleasure as wholehearted attention, Brewer points to a tension inherent in Gandhi's struggle with desire. By attending to his longing, Gandhi found pleasure in desire itself.[10]

Gandhi did not want to enjoy his desire for sensual pleasure. He wanted to transcend it. His approach to other forms of desire was more complicated, however. Even at his most austere, he never rejected the pleasure of good company. It would be tempting to distinguish between the flavor of those mangoes and the joy Gandhi found in his relationship with Chaudhurani. Whereas one pleasure risked the slavery of the senses, the other freed him to enjoy even the absence of the object of his desire. Yet his relationship with Chaudhurani, like his relationship to those mangoes, cannot sustain neat distinctions between bodily slavery and spiritual freedom. Tellingly, he concluded his note to Chaudhurani by pleading with her to come to the ashram to perform domestic labor; in a statement that reeks of sexist paternalism, he explained, "Great and good though you are, you are not a complete woman without achieving the ability to do household work." Gandhi's desire for Chaudhurani's company devolved into an effort to put her in her place. It's worth noting that Gandhi did not look down upon "household work"; on the contrary, he valorized the most "lowly" tasks as acts of spiritual devotion. Gandhi's letter was meant to be light-hearted and playful; he signed "lawgiver," as if to mock his desire for control. In the words of historian Vinay Lal, while Gandhi "appeared to work with a crude conception of what it means to be male or female, his entire life can be read as an attempt to bring us to a new threshold of understanding the notions of masculinity and femininity." Despite such complications, Gandhi's suggestion that Chaudhurani become a "complete woman" through housework displays the desire for control at the heart of his obsession with dietary restraint.[11]

That same day, he wrote Chaudhurani again to share three verses from the Ashtavakra Gita, a classic text in the nondualist Hindu philosophical tradition of Advaika Vedanta. The first verse hinges on an analogy with *amrit*, the nectar of immortality:

> If you aspire after deliverance, my child, give up sense pleasures like
>   poison and
> enjoy forgiveness, straightforwardness, compassion, contentment, and
> truthfulness as you would *amrit*.

Etymologically related to the Greek word *ambrosia*, *amrit* carries the same literal meaning—a liquid that imparts immortality—while also bearing the more general connotation of heavenly flavor we associate with ambrosia. Between the sweetness of the tongue and the sweetness of the soul lies the richness of this passage and of Gandhi's approach to flavor and food. The verse commands us to "enjoy" higher pleasures—not to give up all pleasure. We might conclude that Gandhi's goal was to replace "sense pleasures" with the pleasures of "forgiveness, straightforwardness, compassion, contentment, and truthfulness." But why send such a verse to Chaudhurani the very day he had written to her pining for her company and the joy of shared mangoes? It's as if Gandhi was compelled to share his struggle to overcome sensory desire with the object of that desire.[12]

The following day, Gandhi wrote again with more verses from the Ashtavakra Gita on overcoming the desire for pleasure. Yet he began with a note that teems with the pleasure of desire. "You still continue to haunt me even in my sleep," he told Chaudhurani. "No wonder Panditji calls you the greatest *shakti* of India. You may have cast that spell over him. You are performing the trick over me now. If you are the greatest *shakti*, you will enslave India by becoming her slave in thought, word and deed." The word *shakti* is difficult to translate. The editors of Gandhi's collected works gloss the term as "embodiment of life force." Gandhi clearly meant this as a compliment. Yet there is a distinct ambiguity in his portrayal of Chaudhurani as a sorceress casting spells, entrapping him and enslaving India. It would have been in keeping with his philosophy of *swaraj* if he had charged Chaudhurani with freeing India by becoming her slave. Instead, he declared that she was "enslaving India," by which he really meant that she was enslaving him. Or was it his desire for her that was enslaving him? Regardless of whether he acted on his feelings for Chaudhurani, Gandhi felt, those feelings were rendering him unable to fight for the freedom of India. He was aware that desire need not be fulfilled to be pleasurable, but he found something disquieting—indeed, "enslaving"—in what the philosopher William Desmond calls "desire's infinitude and wholeness." Gandhi hesitated to embrace even his most "pure" desire—perhaps because he could not separate the bodily from the spiritual, perhaps because he remained unconvinced that all bodily pleasures were impure.[13]

Gandhi wrote yet again the following day, May 3, 1920, to send more verses that speak to his spiritual predicament:

> It is strange that even a man abiding in the Supreme Oneness and set on attaining *moksha* should get distraught with passion, yielding to its overmastering urge through experience of the pleasure it brings.

> It is strange that a man who knows for certain that the desire which has possessed him is an enemy of knowledge should yet long for pleasure even though extremely enfeebled and nearing death.

Gandhi knew "for certain" that he should not crave mangoes or the company of a woman, but he continued to "long for pleasure." He returned to an alimentary analogy in order to highlight his challenge: "You will note that the verses in the fourth chapter are somewhat dangerous. It is strong food for a delicate stomach." It is not clear what convinced him that these verses were "somewhat dangerous." Perhaps it was their frank admission of the challenge of overcoming sensual pleasure. One line declares, "None but the man of perfect knowledge has the strength to end all desire and aversion, in all the four planes of existence, from Brahma to a blade of grass." Perhaps Gandhi worried that he would never become "a man of perfect knowledge," that the challenge would be too steep even for him. Perhaps that is why he sent these verses to Chaudhurani. He needed to share his struggle as he had yearned to share those mangoes.[14]

Across decades of dietary experimentation, from the early tests of his vegetarianism to the epic fasts at the end of his life, Gandhi held on to one cardinal rule: he shared his struggles. While he loved to offer advice about food, he also shared his doubts about his diet. At his best, he found in food a form of self-transcendence in service to a larger community. To eat with greater zest and delight, he felt, we must first liberate ourselves from egotistical eating; the more we individualize the pleasures of food, the more we trap ourselves in our bodies. Food should expand our horizons and connect us to others, but it was not primarily eating or even cooking that became for Gandhi a way of connecting. Rather, it was the ambiguities and uncertainties of his diet that inspired him to reach out. It was its imperfection that rendered his diet a source of connection. That is the lesson of the luscious mangoes. Our struggles with food are never ours alone.

EPILOGUE

The Gandhi Diet

Some look upon me as a fool, a crank or a faddist. I must admit that wherever I go I am sought out by fools, cranks and faddists. One can conclude from this that I must be having the characteristics of all these three types.

GANDHI, 1929

W HEN I BEGAN GRADUATE SCHOOL, MY NEW DOCTOR TOLD ME that I should "lose a little weight." I was shocked. I had been an athlete since elementary school, and still played basketball on a regular basis. I never thought about my weight. Unaware, I had gone from a 190-pound athletic young man to a 240-pound not-so-young man. After meeting with my doctor, I started to exercise more, but did not change my diet. I lost a few pounds, but they did not stay off. Gandhi's example led me to a more systematic change in how I approached food.

I still struggle with my diet and, in particular, with eating too much. I often prepare too much food, and then feel compelled to finish everything on my plate. Having two small children has only increased my culinary challenges; now, I find myself finishing their food as well as my own. Writing this book helped me think through particular nutritional questions—how much salt I should eat, for example—but the more important lessons I took from my research concern the danger of compulsive behavior. Whereas Gandhi was obsessed with limiting his food intake, I often bring a similar obsession to finishing food.

I was tempted to call this book *The Gandhi Diet*. Originally, I envisioned it as a series of practical insights gleaned from Gandhi's approach to salt, vegetarianism, sweets, whole foods, raw foods, and fasting. The more I studied Gandhi's relationship to food, the more I realized my approach to that relationship was fundamentally wrong. I was probing a man's life for lessons about what to eat, rather than studying what he ate for lessons about how to live. It was foolish, I realized, to repackage Gandhi's diet as a series of simple maxims about food or nutrition. The Salt March was not about the dangers of sodium. The controversy surrounding mealie pap has much to teach us, none of it about the nutritional value of corn. If I ignored the social, the political, and the religious, I would obscure all that was most essential to Gandhi's life with food.

I came to look with suspicion upon the very idea of drawing lessons from Gandhi's constantly evolving, remarkably complex relationship with food. It would be impossible to render Gandhi's diet a "model" anyone would want to follow—or could, even if they tried. Despite constantly publicizing his dietary experiments and offering advice to anyone who would listen, Gandhi failed to convince most of his contemporaries to follow his dietary example. Many Indians saw his dietary experiments as too strange to emulate. One public figure wrote privately of the mahatma, "Queer food he eats; only fruit and nuts. No salt: milk, ghee, etc. being animal products, avoided religiously. No fire should be necessary in the making of the food, fire being unnatural." Others criticized Gandhi publicly. The prominent communist E. M. S. Namboodiripad mocked his participation in the London Vegetarian Society and offered a comparison with another famous radical: "While Gandhi, the young barrister, was writing articles for the *Vegetarian*, Lenin, also a young lawyer, was translating Marx, Sydney Webb, etc. and himself writing *The Development of Capitalism in Russia*. Lenin combined the militant mass movement of the working class with the most advanced ideology. Gandhi combined it with the most reactionary and obscurantist of ideologies that was current in the contemporary world." Namboodiripad overlooked the fact that vegetarianism was radical in Victorian England, and that many of Gandhi's vegetarian friends were revolutionary in more ways than their diet. Yet he was right to question the relationship between Gandhi's diet and his politics. A powerful force in Gandhi's own life, his diet failed to attract a large following even among his closest supporters.[1]

Gandhi knew that his diet struck others as odd. "Among my fads," he admitted in 1929, "is the one concerning experiments in diet." The peculiar "crankiness" of his eccentric relationship with food complicates any effort to reduce his dietary choices to facile lessons on what we should eat. Indeed, one of the most important lessons we can take from him is to be suspicious of such prescriptions, especially when they are divorced from the ethical and political questions he so consistently linked to his diet.[2]

Take, for example, his fasts. Fasting is trendy. Look through the diet shelf of your local bookstore, and you will find many titles that promote the power of caloric restriction. Whether they suggest that you "feast for five days, fast for two" or pursue more gradual ways to "turn on your 'skinny gene,'" most books that promote fasting focus on the body. For Gandhi, fasting was a way to grow spiritually—and to fight injustice—not just a way to improve his health. In today's world, over a billion people suffer chronic hunger. Some 3.5 million children die as a result of hunger-related illness every year. In the United States, almost fifty million people do not get enough to eat each day. It is their suffering we must end if we wish to honor Gandhi's legacy.[3]

Gandhi's life reveals the power of connecting food to the struggle for justice. Learning the most important lessons from Gandhi's diet requires pushing beyond questions of nutrition to the larger social and political impact of what we eat, how we eat, and how we live. Without concerted action, the raw, organic, and unprocessed foods Gandhi savored will remain just another elite luxury. Many scholars have championed food democracy—defined, in the words of Neva Hassanein, as "the idea that people can and should be actively participating in shaping the food system." Gandhi's history validates that basic idea, while offering a more expansive understanding of food democracy as the ways in which attention to diet and agriculture can empower the struggle against racism, imperialism, and other antidemocratic forces. As the anthropologist Mary Douglas wrote, "The ordered system which is a meal represents all the ordered systems associated with it." Mealie pap, for example, was bound up with the racism of the white South African authorities, as well as the class and caste politics of Gandhi and his fellow prisoners. If he had never evolved in his relationship to that dish, his dietary politics would demonstrate the limitations of racial and culinary borders. By connecting his culinary cosmopolitanism to his burgeoning antiracist and anti-imperial politics, Gandhi offered a radical vision of food democracy.[4]

Gandhi strove to resolve the greatest paradox confronting the modern world: many people starve, while others eat too much. His austerity was a direct response to the deprivation of India's poor. "In India we have got three millions of people having to be satisfied with one meal a day," he wrote. "You and I have no right to anything that we really have until these three million are clothed and fed better." Farmers produce enough food for everyone. The problem is that we do not know how to share. In Gandhi's words, "Whatever we eat after our hunger has been satisfied is stolen food." It is vital that we not overlook his overly romantic conception of agriculture or his inability to confront the vast inequality in land distribution that underpins rural poverty in much of the world. Still, it would be a missed opportunity to ignore the lessons we might take from Gandhi's long engagement with rural development and his insistence on the fundamental oneness of the agricultural economy. He recognized that a healthy diet requires healthy food, and that what people eat depends upon the political, economic, and ecological networks that decide what kind of food is available and at what cost. He pioneered a sustainable approach to agriculture built around small farmers providing for their local communities—farmers like Shankar Rao.[5]

I met Mr. Rao at his farm in the winter of 2013. He greeted me cautiously, smiling only after we began talking about the progress of his crops. Rao supports a family of four on just 1.25 acres of land. His village, Bodad, lies in a remote, hilly region a few hours from Gandhi's ashram. The nearby jungles harbor monkeys, tigers, and the blue bull, an antelope notorious for raiding farmers' fields. Even more threatening than the blue bull, the risk of drought stalks these isolated hills. Without any source of irrigation, most families depend on the rain to water their crops. I visited Bodad in the dry season, when most farms were brown with thirst. Rao's fields, by contrast, were an oasis of green. To understand his success requires learning about more than water management, crop diversification, and natural pesticides. It requires seeing the relationship between food and the earth as Gandhi saw it—a seamless ecological whole.

Rao's biggest challenge is an erratic supply of water. During the monsoon, his farm is pounded with rain. For years, the vast majority of rainwater ran off the land rather than soaking into the soil. Such monsoon runoff was a double loss; it failed to recharge wells, and eroded vital soil and nutrients. To stop such losses, Rao dug a farm pond—a square hole, roughly forty feet by forty feet and some twenty feet deep. Now, when the rains come, much of the water stays on the land, where it seeps slowly into the ground, recharging the family well.

Greater access to water could not alone have freed Rao's family from poverty. To achieve economic stability, he began to cultivate a range of fruits and vegetables. Tomatoes, onions, mangoes, papayas—many of the new crops are eaten directly by the family. The rich variety of their fields translates into more nutritious meals. Healthy farms mean more produce for the community, and more money and better health for farmers. After every harvest, Rao brings some of his fruit crop to a nearby village. In his first season, he was able to sell enough papayas to turn his farm into a profitable enterprise.

Rao's family received support from the Kamalnayan Jamnalal Bajaj Foundation, a large rural development NGO that works to implement a Gandhian approach to community development. Jamnalal Bajaj, one of India's most successful industrialists, gave Gandhi the land to build his last ashram. The Bajaj family continues to support villagers throughout the region, including farmers like Rao. The Bajaj Foundation supports water conservation practices, women's collaboratives, alternative energy systems, and sustainable agriculture. The foundation also provides farmers with seeds and training to plant *vadis*—the same kind of small-scale fruit and vegetable gardens Gandhi praised. *Vadis* do not create a fair banking system or fully protect farmers from the vagaries of the market, but they do provide an alternative source of income and a diverse supply of fresh fruits and vegetables.

Gandhi believed food could be the foundation of a more just world, and he fought to end the inequality that defined the global food system. He failed. In the Indian state of Maharashtra, home to Gandhi's last ashram and Shankar Rao's farm, over fifty thousand farmers have killed themselves in the last two decades. These deaths are only the most visible sign of a widespread distress that haunts farming communities throughout the world. From the fields of India to the vast farms of California, those who grow our food receive only a tiny fraction of the value of the crops they produce. In what must be the cruelest paradox of the modern era, many of the people who grow the world's food cannot afford a sufficiently varied diet to prevent malnutrition. Children and pregnant women often suffer the most. The terror of hunger drives the rural poor into cities, overflowing crowded slums from Lima and Bangkok to Jakarta and Mumbai.[6]

Our challenge is to learn from the success of individuals like Shankar Rao and organizations like the Bajaj Foundation while struggling to transform the larger systems that perpetuate inequality. As Gandhi demonstrated, there is power in connecting small-scale innovation with large-scale social movements. The scale of the problems facing our world—from environmental collapse to rising inequality—requires the kind of ambition Gandhi brought to all his efforts, an ambition that could devolve into imperial coercion but that, at its best, was tempered by compassion and humility.

Gandhi's humility inspired him to be tolerant of difference. Although he believed deeply in his dietary principles, he respected the right of others to disagree. "I heartily dislike drinking, meat-eating and smoking," he wrote, "but I tolerate all these in Hindus, Mohammedans and Christians even as I expect them to tolerate my abstinence." An advocate of nonviolence should never "force the other to his view." When Gandhi criticized those who spent money on tea rather than feeding their families, some of his most zealous followers responded by forcibly shuttering tea shops. Gandhi acted swiftly to rein in his errant disciples. "I would not like to have even the best thing done under compulsion," he wrote. As we have seen, Gandhi's tolerance of beef eaters remains tragically relevant in an India in which the protection of the cow, a cause Gandhi held dear, is used as a pretext for violence against religious minorities and other vulnerable communities.[7]

For Gandhi, rejecting meat meant rejecting the ego. Where an extremist would ignore the middle ground, Gandhi pursued a pragmatic approach to protecting animals from slaughter. In 1921, he penned an open letter to the Parsis, a large religious community in India that does not forbid meat eating. "I myself never eat meat," Gandhi began. "I am not asking Parsi men and women to become vegetarians," he explained, but to "avoid an excess" of meat. Although Gandhi believed that it was wrong to eat even small amounts of meat, he recognized that sometimes more good would be accomplished by encouraging moderation than by demanding complete abstention. That lesson has recently found surprising advocates.[8]

In November 2013, the Norwegian Army launched a remarkably Gandhian assault at the Rena military base some ninety miles north of Oslo. Their target was global warming; their weapon of choice, the soy taco. Inspired by an international campaign to lower greenhouse gas emissions by reducing meat consumption, the army had decided to institute a meat-free day every week. The brainchild of a savvy advertising executive, Sid Lerner, the "meat-free Monday" campaign was ten years old by the time it reached the Norwegian Army. In the United States, the movement's roots go back to food rationing during the First World War. In 2003, Lerner and his colleagues launched a public relations campaign to convince people to give up meat—at least for one day a week. The campaign galvanized people looking to eat less meat but unwilling to become full-time vegetarians, people sometimes known as flexitarians, reducetarians, or "vegans before six" (VB6). No matter what we call it, a movement has begun that has changed the conversation about how to eat ethically and responsibly. A partnership between those who want to eat meat ethically and those who believe it is never ethical to eat meat, this coalition has demonstrated the power of tolerance as a movement-building strategy.[9]

Even if he knew an animal had been well treated, Gandhi still would not eat it. He did, however, recognize degrees of injustice, and focused on the most egregious cruelty toward animals. Such distinctions have become a major industry. While consumers pay extra for cage-free eggs and humanely raised meat, a variety of rating systems attempt to evaluate the quality of life of the animals before they are killed. Such systems often obscure as much as they reveal; savvy consumers have grown wary of "cage-free eggs" produced by chickens that live their entire lives in cramped barns. Major disagreements divide those who believe it is never right to eat meat and those who strive to eat meat in ways that are compassionate. Both groups are, however, part of the same minority that endeavors to prevent animal suffering and end the brutality of the meat industry.[10]

Gandhi would have been delighted by the movement to end the suffering of animals. In 2008, California voters banned the confinement of farm animals in cages that do not allow them to "turn around freely, lie down, stand up or fully extend their limbs." Many consumers are familiar with cage-free eggs, but most have never been inside a factory farm; they have never seen row after row of chickens crowded into battery cages without room to turn around or spread their wings. The new law was thus a triumph of the imagination. Everyone agreed the law would raise the cost of eggs. Voters approved it anyway, proving that people are capable of caring for animals they have never seen.[11]

Such radical empathy was at the heart of Gandhi's vegetarianism and his diet. Like him, many of today's most prominent vegetarian authors and organizations combine an emphasis on personal health with a commitment to the welfare of animals and the environment. In the words of sociologist Donna Maurer, "For many vegetarians—and particularly for organization leaders—'being' a vegetarian is not a static state; it is a process of 'becoming' through shifting personal motivations and increasing degrees of commitment." Such a process of becoming marked all of Gandhi's dietary commitments. He continually struggled to refine and deepen his dietary values and practices, even while remaining open to learning from those whose diets were categorically different from his own.[12]

From his early years in London to the last months of his life, Gandhi explored the culinary traditions of the world. He encountered many of his favorite dishes in the Gujarati kitchens of his youth. But even his most "Indian" comfort foods demonstrate how culinary traditions were shaped by global circuits of exchange and innovation. Recognizing the achievements of his culinary cosmopolitanism should not entail overlooking its limitations, nor the degree to which his peculiar dietary experiments were made possible by his class status. Historian Camille Bégin has noted a shift in food studies literature from "the notion of culinary cosmopolitanism typically used to describe the middle-class and elite urban restaurant scene" to a greater appreciation for "widespread, working-class, localized cosmopolitanisms." Nevertheless, we must continue to recognize, in the words of sociologists Josée Johnston and Shyon Baumann, that "culinary cosmopolitanism occurs in a context of grossly maldistributed power and resources rendering those in the geo-political core of the world system tremendously privileged." At some point, culinary cosmopolitanism becomes culinary imperialism. In Gandhi's case, class status was rivaled by the mobility shaped by those circuits of imperial labor that brought together the Indian and African diasporas—not just in Africa itself, but in the Caribbean, the Americas, Europe, and elsewhere.[13]

In Gandhi's diet, the homogenizing tendencies of globalization intersected with the diversifying consequences of the migratory flows created by empire. As the geographers Robyn Longhurst and Lynda Johnston have stated, "The notion of culinary cosmopolitanism is also complicated by enmeshed bodies and places." Gandhi's diet spanned the borders of nations and of religions. While there was something distinctly Jain and Hindu about his spiritual outlook on food, Gandhi also learned from Christian and Muslim approaches to diet. His religious pluralism informed his culinary cosmopolitanism. The reverse was also true: his adventures in eating helped him to respect other religious traditions. His diet contributed to what Debjani Ganguly has called Gandhi's "moral internationalism based on the notion of compassion for and connectivity with strangers."[14]

The relationship between his faith and his food helps to explain why Gandhi invested so heavily in matters of diet. He cared about what he ate because he saw eating as a religious act; his body was a tool for doing God's work. When a Danish missionary fell ill at Gandhi's ashram, he prepared her a detailed diet: "You may take milk in the morning with some fruit and bread and *dahi* [yogurt] in rice for breakfast, with some vegetables simply boiled." Along with this dietary advice, Gandhi offered what he called "a wretched sermon" on the spiritual importance of maintaining physical health. "Only you must put your body right even as an artisan's first duty is to keep his tools in order," he wrote. "God has given us this body as a tool to be used efficiently for His service."[15]

Gandhi counseled against making "our stomach our God" and wasting our lives "in its worship." If his love for food at times veered toward worship, it was not his stomach that deserves blame; his passion for food was inspired by a belief in the transformative power of diet. In 1914, he asked a close relative, "Why should we experiment with food? Where will it take us?" Gandhi's answer made clear that a new diet should lead to a new world. When we revise what we eat, he explained, "We are setting up everything new." By recognizing the fundamental significance of food, he revealed why diets can be so painful and so often lead to failure. "Our normal food is full of rituals," he explained—rituals that easily become habits. "To cling to that food," he declared, "is attachment."

When it came to avoiding dietary attachment, he did not distinguish between "good" and "bad" ways of eating. All diets, even the most healthy, have the capacity to become attachments.[16]

While Gandhi pressured his family, friends, and followers to learn from his dietary experiments, he did not push anyone to copy his diet entirely. He knew that no one diet works for all people. Not only do "habits differ from nation to nation," he explained, but "the same item of food affects different individuals differently." Gandhi rejected what he called a "dogmatic" approach to diet. He was dogmatic when it came to the religious facets of his diet, especially his vegetarianism—but most of his key dietary principles, such as avoiding salt or eating vegetables raw, were the result of extended experimentation. Rather than obediently following a Gandhi diet, our goal should be to learn from Gandhi's dietary experiments how to guide our own.[17]

Forging a healthy lifestyle was, in Gandhi's words, "a process without end." Within the science of nutrition, he wrote, "Every day new facts are observed and new ideas emerge." What sociologist Claude Fischler calls "nutritional cacophony" leads many people to turn away from the idea of eating well. Others put undue faith in whatever nutritional advice happens to be trendy. Gandhi charted a middle ground between nutritional apathy and blind devotion to the latest nutritional findings. He assessed each dietary question in the light of expert advice as well as his own experience. From how much salt to consume to the advantages of raw food, Gandhi revised his habits in accordance with new evidence. The psychoanalyst Erik Erikson declared that Gandhi's "preoccupation with food" was "obsessive and faddish." Gandhi's relationship to food was, at times, obsessive, and as we have seen, Gandhi himself laughed at the "faddish" nature of his diet. But dismissing his diet because it was "faddish" would require equating all new ideas with groundless "fads," and ignoring the benefits of dietary curiosity.[18]

Today, many key elements of Gandhi's diet are undergoing a renaissance. From raw food to whole grains, his choices are increasingly popular. What would most delight the mahatma is the growing movement to link food to the social and economic empowerment of the poor and to the health of the planet. Gandhi strove to transform the global food system and eliminate its colonial inequalities. His mission lives on wherever people care about the ethical and ecological consequences of what they eat. By exploring his diet, we can discover how to connect what we eat to our deepest values. Only then will our diets become about more than ourselves. There are many ways to begin. Gandhi's service took the form of salt marches and epic fasts, but also of homemade almond milk, fresh fig salad, and the joy of sharing mangoes with a friend.

Recipes from Gandhi's Diet

The following recipes are adapted from meals created by Gandhi or are based on key principles of his diet. Several are staples in my family.

....

BREAKFAST CRUNCH

My favorite breakfast recipe, this delicious, crunchy dish combines three of Gandhi's favorite foods: yogurt, nuts, and fruit.

1 small apple
1 cup plain yogurt
2 tablespoons nut butter (peanut butter or almond butter)
½ cup granola

Dice the apple and mix with the yogurt and the nut butter. Sprinkle the granola on top.

LUNI SALAD

A nice alternative to lettuce, luni *(purslane) packs a mild lemony taste along with one of the highest concentrations of heart-healthy omega-3 fats you can find in a plant. Increasingly available in farmers' markets,* luni *can also be found in Chinese or Mexican groceries. But before you go to the store, check your backyard. You might have* luni *already.*

    2 cups *luni* (purslane)
    1 cup cherry tomatoes
    1 apple
    1 tablespoon sunflower seeds
    ½ cup raw pecans

Wash and dry the *luni* and tear large leaves into bite-sized pieces. Slice the tomatoes in half and dice the apple. Combine the *luni*, tomatoes, apple, sunflower seeds, and pecans.

SIMPLE FRUIT SALAD

Gandhi sent this recipe in a letter to a friend. He used sweet limes rather than grapes and apple, but sweet limes are hard to find outside of India. He also included a pinch of salt, a rare move on his part that I have found unnecessary to replicate. The secret of this recipe is that fruit salad does not need elaborate, sugary dressing. A little bit of pomegranate juice adds a tangy depth.

    2 oranges
    1 bunch red grapes, halved
    1 apple (Fuji or similar), diced
    ¼ cup pomegranate juice

Peel the oranges and mix their segments with the grapes and the diced apple. Pour the pomegranate juice over the fruit mixture.

ALMOND MILK AND ALMOND JELLY

Gandhi labored to perfect his recipe for a "butter-like" almond jelly and an almond milk. Of the jelly, he wrote, "I eat it with vegetables." I like to put the jelly on toast or on top of a diced apple. The almond milk is a nice addition to a smoothie.

    2 cups raw almonds
    Water
    Salt and sugar to taste

Soak the almonds in hot water for approximately one hour. Remove the almond peels and crush the almonds (a food processor or a mortar and pestle both work well). Mix the crushed almonds with 4 ounces of water and boil until the water evaporates. You now have almond jelly. For almond milk, add 2 cups of water and stir briskly over low heat until a milklike consistency is achieved. Add a small amount of salt or sugar to taste.

DATE DELIGHTS

Gandhi rejected desserts as distractions from more fulfilling satisfactions. But his rejection was far from absolute. Goat's milk was a staple of Gandhi's diet. He also frequently ate dates, known for their natural sweetness and rich with fiber and nutrients. Together, the warmed dates and goat's cheese make an amazing treat that can inspire—rather than distract—our better selves.

    1 pound pitted dates
    2 tablespoons goat cheese

Slice the dates in half. Spoon a small amount of goat cheese inside a split date and cover with another date half. Place the stuffed dates on a baking sheet and put in the oven at 300°F for approximately 5 minutes or until the dates and cheese have warmed.

WHEAT BERRY PORRIDGE

Gandhi loved whole wheat and savored his whole wheat berry porridge. He varied how he made the porridge: sometimes, he roasted the wheat berries whole, ground them into a powder, then soaked the powder in water and milk for 10 minutes. I find method described here easier. For a sweeter porridge, consider adding dried fruit or a drizzle of maple syrup.

    1 cup wheat berries
    2 cups water
    1 cup almond milk
    ¼ cup chopped walnuts
    Cinnamon and salt to taste

Add the wheat berries to the water in a large saucepan. Bring to a boil, cover, and reduce to a simmer. Cook until the water has been absorbed (approximately 40 minutes). Stir in the almond milk and simmer uncovered for 5–10 minutes, stirring occasionally. Add walnuts and cinnamon and salt to taste.

TOMATO *RASAM*

Gandhi believed in the healing qualities of tamarind. I am drawn to its tangy kick. Whether for its nutrition or its taste, tamarind is the key ingredient in rasam, *often called the chicken soup of South India. I prefer eating* rasam *like a soup, but it is also often poured over rice. Gandhi called it South India's "famous* rasam" *and asked a colleague for a recipe so that he could make it himself.*

    1 tsp olive oil
    ¼ tsp black mustard seeds
    2 cloves garlic, diced finely or crushed
    1 tsp roasted cumin (*jeera*), powdered or crushed
    ¼ tsp asafoetida powder
    ¼ tsp turmeric powder

3 ripe medium-sized tomatoes, diced
3 cups water
2 tsp tamarind paste
Salt and black pepper to taste
¼ cup chopped coriander leaves

In a large saucepan, heat the olive oil over medium heat (high heat will damage the oil) and add the mustard seeds. When they start to pop, add the garlic, cumin, asafoetida, and turmeric. Stir over medium heat for 1–2 minutes and then add the tomatoes. Continue to stir for 2–3 minutes, then add 3 cups of water and the tamarind paste. Stir and continue to simmer for another 5 minutes. Add salt and black pepper to taste, garnish with the coriander leaves, and enjoy.

....

BANANA BISCUITS

6 medium-sized green bananas
1 cup whole wheat flour
2½ teaspoons baking powder
½ teaspoon salt
1 cup almond milk

Peel the green bananas and slice them into small discs. Dry the banana discs (see note below for drying options). Grind the resulting banana chips into flour (a food processor does the job well). Combine the banana flour with the wheat flour, the baking powder, and the salt. Make a well in the flour mixture and pour in the almond milk. Stir until the almond milk is absorbed and the dough comes together. Create small (1-inch) balls of dough and roll on a floured service, then press dough into discs. Place the discs on a baking sheet and bake at 400°F for 15–20 minutes or until the biscuits have just turned gold on top.

Note: If you decide, like Gandhi, to make your own banana chips, you have three options. You could put the banana discs in the oven for a few hours at the lowest possible temperature, turning them at least once. You could buy a dehydrator. Or you could follow Gandhi in using the power of the sun. For a simpler recipe, consider buying ready-made banana chips. Another way to simplify the recipe is to eat the uncooked banana powder (sans wheat flour and baking powder) along with dried mangoes, as Gandhi did. That mixture is not the same as a warm biscuit, but it is still delicious.

Notes

INTRODUCTION: THE SCALE

Epigraph: Gandhi, *The Good Boatman*, 445.

1 Nanda, *In Search of Gandhi*, 229.

2 Many biographies of Gandhi mention his obsession with food, but only a few examine that obsession in any detail. The most thorough studies include Alter, *Gandhi's Body*, and Roy, *Alimentary Tracts*.

3 Pollan, *In Defense of Food*, 1.

4 Eck, *Darśan*; Amin, "Gandhi as Mahatma"; and Herman, *Gandhi and Churchill*, 359.

5 Mahatma Gandhi, "General Knowledge about Health, XXXII," *Indian Opinion*, August 9, 1913, in the electronic version of *The Collected Works of Mahatma Gandhi* (*CWMG*). In the pages that follow, all citations without a stated author were written by Gandhi and are included in the *CWMG*. Despite its ease of use, there are significant problems with the electronic version of the *CWMG*; the most complete and authoritative version of the *CWMG* remains the original printed version.

6 Cannon and Leitzmann, "The New Nutrition Science Project"; Schubert et al., "Re-imagining the 'Social' in the Nutrition Sciences"; and Gottlieb and Joshi, *Food Justice*.

7 Bilgrami, "Gandhi's Integrity," 79.

8 Many books aim to guide readers toward a more compassionate and politically engaged relationship to food. See Holt-Giménez, *Food Movements Unite!*; Alkon and Agyeman, *Cultivating Food Justice*; Guthman, *Weighing In*; Winne, *Food Rebels, Guerrilla Gardeners, and Smart-Cookin' Mamas*; and Salatin, *Everything I Want to Do Is Illegal*.

9 Guha, *Gandhi before India*.

10 Kumar, *Radical Equality*; and Skaria, *Unconditional Equality*.

11　On culinary cosmopolitanism, see Ray, *The Ethnic Restaurateur*; Cappeliez and Johnston, "From Meat and Potatoes to 'Real-Deal' Rotis"; Green, "Kebabs and Port Wine"; Jhala, "Cosmopolitan Kitchens"; and Heldke, *Exotic Appetites*.

12　Mannur, *Culinary Fictions*, 204; Narayan, *Dislocating Cultures*, 178–80; and Black, "Recipes for Cosmopolitanism," 2.

13　Gandhi, *An Autobiography*, 132; and "General Knowledge about Health, IX," *Indian Opinion*, March 1, 1913. Also see Jordens, *Gandhi's Religion*.

14　Scrinis, Nutritionism, 9.

15　"General Knowledge about Health, XI," *Indian Opinion*, April 5, 1913; and "General Knowledge about Health, IX," *Indian Opinion*, March 1, 1913.

16　"Letter to Maganlal Gandhi," about 1914; and Arnold, *Decoding Anorexia*.

17　"Letter to Hermann Kallenbach," October 22, 1911.

18　"Fragment of Letter to Manilal and Jamnadas Gandhi," Saturday on or after June 13, 1914.

CHAPTER 1: SALT

Epigraph: "Speech at Prayer Meeting," before March 9, 1930.

1　"Salt Tax," *Young India*, February 27, 1930; Kurlansky, *Salt*, 63; and Laszlo, *Salt*.

2　"History of Salt Manufacture," February 27, 1930. Also see Dutt, *The Economic History of India in the Victorian Age*, 143–56; Rothermund, *An Economic History of India*, 92–93 and 102–3; and Moxham, "Salt Starvation in British India."

3　"Notes," *Young India*, April 3, 1930; Bondurant, *Conquest of Violence*, 88–101; and Dalton, *Mahatma Gandhi*, chapter 4.

4　Sifferlin, "Salt Sugar Fat." Also see Moss, *Salt, Sugar, Fat*.

5　"Letter to Shankarlal Banker," September 7, 1918.

6　"The Doom of Purdah," *Young India*, June 28, 1928; and "Implications of Constructive Program," *Harijan*, August 18, 1940. Also see Vajpeyi, *Righteous Republic*; and Rathore, *Indian Political Theory*.

7　"Letter to Jawaharlal Nehru," March 11, 1930; and "Letter to Satin D. Gupta," *Bombay Chronicle*, March 10, 1930.

8　"Letter to Manibehn Patel," March 9, 1930; "Speech at Prayer Meeting," March 10, 1930; and "Speech at Prayer Meeting," before March 9, 1930.

9　Guthman, "Commentary on Teaching Food," 264.

10　"Indian Vegetarians," *Vegetarian*, February 7, 1891; and "The Foods of India," *Vegetarian Messenger*, June 1, 1891.

11　"Salt Tax in India," *Indian Opinion*, July 8, 1905; "Lord Curzon," *Indian Opinion*, August 26, 1905; "The Salt Tax," *Indian Opinion*, October 14, 1905; Gandhi, *Hind Swaraj*, 21 and 98; "Letter to E. L. Sale," June 19, 1919;

"The Death Dance," *Young India*, March 9, 1922; and "Letter to Purushottam-das Thakurdas," October 8, 1929.

12 Gandhi was not the first to target the salt tax. As early as 1844, riots against the tax had erupted in Surat District. See Suchitra, "What Moves Masses." Also see "Interview to a Professor," *Harijan*, May 14, 1938.

13 "Salt Tax," *Young India*, February 27, 1930.

14 On the Raj as prison, see Arnold, "The Colonial Prison." Also see "Letter to Lord Irwin," March 2, 1930; and "Begging the Question," *Young India*, March 12, 1930.

15 Weber, *On the Salt March*, 435.

16 Miller, *I Found No Peace*, 193–99.

17 Lal and DuBois, *A Passionate Life*; Taneja, *Gandhi, Women, and the National Movement*, 133–38; Nanda, *Kamaladevi Chattopadhyay*, 51–54; and Narasimhan, *Kamaladevi Chattopadhyay*, 32–57.

18 Hunt, *Gandhi in London*, 193; "Mr. Churchill on India," *Daily Telegraph*, February 24, 1931; and "Gandhi to Churchill," July 17, 1944.

19 "Meaning of Grinding Poverty," *Young India*, June 11, 1931.

20 "Salt," *Young India*, May 28, 1931; "Letter to Sir George Schuster," March 28, 1934; "Letter to Sir George Schuster," April 14, 1934; "Statement to the Press," November 26, 1934; and Weber, *On the Salt March*, 459.

21 "Interview to H. N. Brailsford," March 17, 1946; "Letter to Lord Wavell," April 6, 1946; "Letter to G. E. B. Abell," May 3, 1946; and "Viceroy's Note on Interview to Gandhiji," April 3 and April 9, 1946.

22 "Note to Vallabhai Patel, Rajendra Prasad, and Jagjivan Ram," September 2, 1946; and "Speech at Prayer Meeting," *Hindustan*, September 3, 1946.

23 *Prarthana Pravachan*, vol. 1, 273–74, CWMG.

24 Gandhi, *Hind Swaraj*, 25.

25 "Remarks at Prayer Meeting, Sabarmati Ashram," March 5, 1930.

26 "Swaraj through Women," *Harijan*, December 2, 1939; "Speech at Prayer Meeting," *Hindustan*, September 3, 1946; "Misrepresentation," *Young India*, March 12, 1930; Kishwar, "Gandhi and Women"; Thapar, "Women as Activists"; and Chatterjee, "1930."

27 "Satyagrahis' March," *Navajivan*, March 9, 1930; "Notes," *Young India*, April 3, 1930; and "Letter to Narandas Gandhi," January 1/6, 1931.

28 "Some Questions," *Young India*, February 20, 1930.

29 "Salt and Cancer," *Young India*, February 27, 1930.

30 Mente et al., "Association of Urinary Sodium and Potassium Excretion with Blood Pressure"; Mozaffarian et al., "Global Sodium Consumption and Death from Cardiovascular Causes"; and O'Donnell et al., "Urinary Sodium and Potassium Excretion, Mortality, and Cardiovascular Events."

31 "Letter to Maganlal Gandhi," March 9, 1911; "Fragment of Letter to Maganlal Gandhi," after November 30, 1910; "Letter to Devdas Gandhi," end of 1917; "Letter to Hermann Kallenbach," April 5, 1911; "Letter to Hermann Kallenbach," April 8, 1911; and "General Knowledge about Health, 13," *Indian Opinion*, March 29, 1913.

32 "Letter to Jamnadas Gandhi," March 29, 1913; "Letter to Jamnadas Gandhi," August 28, 1911; "Letter to Dr. Kulkarni," January 24, 1918; "Letter to Ranchhodlal Patwari," September 9, 1918; "Some Questions," *Navajivan*, September 27, 1925; "Letter to D. Hanumantharao," February 21, 1926; "Letter to Rani Vidyavati," July 15, 1929; and "Unfired Food Experiment," *Young India*, July 18, 1929.

33 "Letter to Prof. Jevons," August 11, 1918; "Speech on Non-Cooperation," December 13, 1920; "Notes," *Young India*, July 17, 1924; "Notes," *Young India*, April 6, 1921; "Belgaum Impressions," *Young India*, January 1, 1925; "Letter to C. Rajagopalachari," March 22, 1924; "Talk to Members of Spinning Club," June 30, 1940; "The Fear of Death," August 14, 1921; "Free Salt for the Salt of the Earth," November 26, 1934; and "Notes," *Young India*, April 3, 1930.

34 "Letter to Budhabhai," November 9, 1930; "Letter to Satis Chandra Das Gupta," May 16, 1931; and "Letter to Narandas Gandhi," September 25/30, 1930.

35 "Letter to Mirabehn," April 8, 1932; "Letter to Mirabehn," June 1, 1932; and "Letter to Brijkrishna Chandiwala," September 11, 1932.

36 "Fragment of Letter to Manilal and Jamnadas Gandhi," Saturday on or after June 13, 1914.

37 Gandhi, *An Autobiography*, 273.

38 "Letter to Munnalal G. Shah," January 28, 1945; Hajari, *Midnight's Furies*; and Khan, *The Great Partition*.

39 "What Is Brahmacharya?" *Young India*, June 5, 1924; Lal, "Nakedness, Nonviolence, and Brahmacharya"; Jordens, *Gandhi's Religion*, 185–98; and Alter, *Gandhi's Body*.

40 "Letter to G. D. Birla," August 17, 1925; "Some Questions," *Navajivan*, September 27, 1925; "Letter to Shambhushanker," August 30, 1926; "Letter to Dr. Kulkarni," January 24, 1918; "Letter to Radhadrishna Bajaj," May 6, 1926; "Letter to Chandrakanta," September 7, 1930; "Letter to Munnalal G. Shah," January 28, 1945; and "Letter to Sumangal Prakash," March 20, 1933.

CHAPTER 2: CHOCOLATE

Epigraph: "Letter to H. S. L. Polak," August 26, 1911.

1 "Letter to H. S. L. Polak," August 26, 1911.

2 "Interview to Margaret Sanger," December 3/4, 1935.

3 "What Is Brahmacharya?" *Young India*, June 5, 1924; and "In Confidence," *Young India*, October 13, 1920.

4 "Interview to Margaret Sanger," December 3/4, 1935; Connelly, *Fatal Misconception*, 99–102; Margaret Sanger Papers Project, "Gandhi and Sanger Debate Love, Lust and Birth Control"; Pokorski, "Sanger and Gandhi"; Sanger, "Does Mr. Gandhi Know Women?"; and Katz, *The Selected Papers of Margaret Sanger*, entries 106 and 115.

5 Mintz, *Tasting Food, Tasting Freedom*, 67–83; Mintz, *Sweetness and Power*; Metcalf, *Imperial Connections*; and Kale, *Fragments of Empire*.

6 Cort, *Jains in the World*, 118–41; Dundas, *The Jains*, 166; Laidlaw, *Riches and Renunciation*; and "General Knowledge about Health [XXXIV]," *Indian Opinion*, August 16, 1913.

7 Mintz, *Tasting Food, Tasting Freedom*, 83.

8 "Letter to Ramdas Gandhi and Family," January 19, 1940; and "Johannesburg Letter," *Indian Opinion*, July 28, 1908.

9 "Madras Tour," *Navajivan*, August 29, 1920; and "Letter to Mahadev Desai," August 7, 1921.

10 "The Foods of India," *Vegetarian Messenger*, June 1, 1891.

11 Elwood, *Narrative of a Journey Overland from England*, 388; "London Gets Mangoes by Air," *New York Times*, August 30, 1931; and Sharma, "Food and Empire."

12 "Letter to Dr. J. Oldfield," October 26, 1906; "Indian Vegetarians—II," *The Vegetarian*, February 14, 1891; "The Foods of India," *Vegetarian Messenger*, June 1, 1891.

13 "Guide to London," most likely written in 1893 and 1894.

14 "My Gaol Experiences [II]," *Indian Opinion*, March 21, 1908; "My Experience in Gaol [III]," *Indian Opinion*, March 21, 1908; and "Starvation of Passive Resisters," *Indian Opinion*, February 26, 1910.

15 Veit, *Modern Food, Moral Food*, 4; "My Gaol Experiences [II]," *Indian Opinion*, March 21, 1908; "My Experience in Gaol [III]," *Indian Opinion*, March 21, 1908; and "My Second Experience in Gaol," *Indian Opinion*, January 2, 1909.

16 "Who Can Go to Gaol?" *Indian Opinion*, June 5, 1909.

17 "My Experience in Gaol [III]," *Indian Opinion*, March 21, 1908; and Slate, "From Mealie Pap to Peanut Milk."

18 Hobart, "A 'Queer-Looking Compound'"; and "My Gaol Experiences [I]," March 7, 1908.

19 On culinary nostalgia, see Sen, "Food, Place, and Memory"; and Swislocki, *Culinary Nostalgia*.

20 "The Plague Panic in South Africa," *Times of India*, April 22, 1899; "My Gaol Experiences [I]," March 7, 1908; "My Gaol Experiences [II]," *Indian Opinion*, March 21, 1908; and "Interview to D. A. Rees," before March 26, 1908.

21 "Petition to Director of Prisons," January 21, 1908; "My Gaol Experiences [I]," March 7, 1908; and "Interview to D. A. Rees," before March 26, 1908.

22 "My Experience in Gaol [III]," *Indian Opinion*, March 21, 1908; and "Johannesburg Letter," undated but completed September 23, 1908.

23 "My Experience in Gaol [III]," *Indian Opinion*, March 21, 1908; "Johannesburg Letter," before July 2, 1908; and "Johannesburg Letter," August 1, 1908.

24 "Letter to the *Transvaal Leader*," August 8, 1908.

25 Gandhi's critics often understate the evolution of Gandhi's views on race, an evolution tied to his changing views on diet; see, for example, Desai and Vahed, *The South African Gandhi*. Also see Banerjee, *Becoming Imperial Citizens*; Guha, *Gandhi before India*; Bhana and Vahed, *The Making of a Political Reformer*; and Swan, *Gandhi*.

26 Gandhi, "The Kaffirs of Natal," *Indian Opinion*, September 2, 1905; Hunt, "Gandhi and the Black People of South Africa"; *Indian Opinion*, February 10, 1912, quoted in Nauriya, *The African Element in Gandhi*; and Slate, *Colored Cosmopolitanism*, 24.

27 "My Second Experience in Gaol," *Indian Opinion*, January 2, 1909; and Guha, *Gandhi before India*, 398.

28 Slate, *Colored Cosmopolitanism*; and "General Knowledge about Health [X]," *Indian Opinion*, March 8, 1913.

29 "Phoenix School," *Indian Opinion*, January 9, 1909.

30 Gandhi, *An Autobiography*, 127–29.

31 "Report of Protector of Indentured Labourers," *Indian Opinion*, August 27, 1910; and Mintz, *Tasting Food, Tasting Freedom*, 72.

32 "Phoenix School," *Indian Opinion*, January 9, 1909; "Letter to H. S. L. Polak," August 26, 1911; "Report of Protector of Indentured Labourers," *Indian Opinion*, August 27, 1910; and "General Knowledge about Health [X]," *Indian Opinion*, March 8, 1913.

33 Crosby, *The Columbian Exchange*; and Norton, "Tasting Empire."

34 Nayar, *Packaging Life*, 173.

35 Garcia, *From the Jaws of Victory*; Bardacke, *Trampling Out the Vintage*; and Pawel, *The Union of Their Dreams*.

36 "Letter to Colonial Secretary," February 22, 1900; Guha, *Gandhi before India*, 275; and Desai and Vahed, *The South African Gandhi*, 56.

37 For an incisive analysis of a major global commodity chain, see Soluri, *Banana Cultures*. Also see "General Knowledge about Health [X]," *Indian Opinion*, March 8, 1913.

38 "Deputation's Voyage," before July 9, 1909.

39 "Deputation's Voyage," before July 9, 1909. Also see Chatterjee, *A Time for Tea*.

40 "General Knowledge about Health, IX," *Indian Opinion*, March 1, 1913; and "My Second Experience in Gaol," *Indian Opinion*, January 2, 1909.

41 Levenstein, *Revolution at the Table*, 93–97; and Anonymous, *An Essay on Tea, Sugar, White Bread and Butter, Country Alehouses, Strong Beer and Geneva, and Other Modern Luxuries.*

42 Vivekananda, "Inspired Talks."

43 Krondi, "The Sweetshops of Kolkata."

44 "Letter to Benarsidas Chaturvedi," September 16, 1945; and "Fragment of Letter to Maganlal Gandhi," after November 30, 1910.

45 "Interview to Journalists," March 6, 1931. Also see Gandhi, *Hind Swaraj*; Vajpeyi, *Righteous Republic*; and Rathore, *Indian Political Theory.*

46 Imprisoned in the Aga Khan's palace from 1942 to 1944, Gandhi penned a series of lessons on health. He wrote them in Gujarati and asked his physician and personal secretary, Dr. Sushila Nayar, to translate them into Hindustani and English. Gandhi himself edited the translations, but they were not published together until after his death in 1948. At that time, they were edited by Jitendra T. Desai and given the title *Key to Health* (Ahmedabad: Navajivan Press, 1948). These writings were reproduced in the CWMG, and it is that version that I consulted in writing this text and that I will cite throughout. To aid the reader, I will provide the chapter headings for each citation, as these are common to both the text printed by Navajivan and the version reproduced in the CWMG. I will use the primary date provided in the CWMG—December 18, 1942—the final date in the Gujarati original. "Food," in *Key to Health*, December 18, 1942. Also see "Speech on 'Ashram Vows' at YMCA, Madras," February 16, 1916; "Unfired Food Experiment," *Young India*, July 18, 1929; "Village Worker's Questions," *Harijan*, May 11, 1935; de la Peña, *Empty Pleasures*; and "Letter to Maganlal Gandhi," October 25, 1914.

47 "Letter to Lakshmi D. Dafda," November 27, 1932; "My Gaol Experiences [II]," *Indian Opinion*, March 21, 1908; "My Experience in Gaol [III]," *Indian Opinion*, March 21, 1908; "My Second Experience in Gaol," *Indian Opinion*, January 2, 1909; "Who Can Go to Gaol?" *Indian Opinion*, June 5, 1909; and "Food," in *Key to Health*, December 18, 1942.

48 "Letter to Mirabehn," June 1, 1932; and "Food," in *Key to Health*, December 18, 1942.

49 Kaelber, "'Tapas,' Birth, and Spiritual Rebirth in the Veda"; Cort, "Singing the Glory of Asceticism"; and Dundas, *The Jains*, 15–16 and 166.

50 "Letter to Shankarlal on 'Ideas about Satyagraha,'" September 2, 1917; "Who May Be Deported," *Indian Opinion*, February 4, 1914; "Speech on Cow Protection, Bettiah," about October 9, 1917; "Speech to Ahmedabad Mill-Hands," Marsh 15, 1918; "Speech at Ras," April 18, 1918; and "Discussion with Heads of Department, Santiniketan," December 19, 1945.

51 "Letter to Tangai Menon," February 23, 1933.

52 "A Talk," April 7, 1947; "General Knowledge about Health [XIII]," *Indian Opinion*, March 29, 1913; and "Food," in *Key to Health*, December 18, 1942.

53 "Speech on 'Ashram Vows' at YMCA, Madras," February 16, 1916; and "Discussion on Boycott at AICC Meeting," *Navajivan*, September 11, 1921.

54 Stiglitz, *The Price of Inequality*, 288; and Singer, *The Most Good You Can Do*.

55 "Letter to Vallabhai Patel," April 18, 1934.

56 "Speech at Prayer Meeting," January 8, 1947; and Guha, *Gandhi before India*, 53.

57 "Letter to Jamnadas Gandhi," August 7, 1913; and "Letter to Jamnadas Gandhi," January 18, 1918.

58 "Speech on 'Ashram Vows' at YMCA, Madras," February 16, 1916; "Draft Constitution for the Ashram," before May 20, 1915; and "Who Can Go to Gaol?" *Indian Opinion*, June 5, 1909.

59 Roy, *Alimentary Tracts*, 114.

60 "Speech on 'Ashram Vows' at YMCA, Madras," February 16, 1916; Belasco and Scranton, *Food Nations*; Nestle, *Food Politics*; Moss, *Salt, Sugar, Fat*; and Winson, *The Industrial Diet*.

CHAPTER 3: GOAT MEAT AND PEANUT MILK

Epigraph: Gandhi, *An Autobiography*, 18.

1 Gandhi, *An Autobiography*, 19.

2 *Natal Advertiser*, February 1, 1895.

3 Gandhi, *An Autobiography*, 47–49, 227–228, and 378.

4 See Shprintzen, *The Vegetarian Crusade*; Preece, *Sins of the Flesh*; Stuart, *The Bloodless Revolution*; Spencer, *Vegetarianism*; Iacobbo and Iacobbo, *Vegetarian America*; and Dombrowski, *The Philosophy of Vegetarianism*.

5 "General Knowledge about Health [XI]," *Indian Opinion*, March 15, 1913; "General Knowledge about Health [XIII]," *Indian Opinion*, March 29, 1913; and "Food," in *Key to Health*, December 18, 1942.

6 Kingsford, *The Perfect Way in Diet*, 1–15.

7 For an example of a polemical debate, see Cordain and Campbell, "The Protein Debate." Also see "Guide to London," 1893–1894; "Letter to Mrs. A. M. Lewis," August 4, 1894; "Books for Sale," *Natal Mercury*, November 28, 1894; "Speech at Meeting of Christians," August 4, 1925; "Letter to Mathuradas Trikumji," May 14, 1927; and "Vegetarianism in Natal," *Vegetarian*, December 21, 1895.

8 "Fragment of Letter to Devdas Gandhi," September 9, 1918; "Letter to K. P. Padmanabha Iyer," July 21, 1927; and "Letter to Chhaganlal Joshi," December 10, 1928.

9 McCay, *The Protein Element in Nutrition*, 184.

10 "Unfired Food Experiment," *Young India*, July 18, 1929.

11 "Unfired Food," *Young India*, August 15, 1929.

12 "To the Editor," *Natal Mercury*, February 4, 1896.

13 "Speech at Meeting of London Vegetarian Society," November 20, 1931.

14 "Letter to the *Natal Mercury*," February 3, 1896; Long, *Jainism*; Chapple, *Jainism and Ecology*; and Cort, *Jains in the World*.

15 "To the Editor," *Natal Mercury*, February 4, 1896; and Oldfield, "My Friend Gandhi."

16 "Interview to the *Vegetarian*—II", *Vegetarian*, June 20, 1891; and Gandhi, *An Autobiography*, 41.

17 "Interview to the *Vegetarian*—II", *Vegetarian*, June 20, 1891; Guha, *Gandhi before India*, 41; Salt, *Animals' Rights*, 90; Hendrick, *Henry Salt*; and Hendrick and Hendrick, *The Savour of Salt*, 25–28.

18 Gregory, *Of Victorians and Vegetarians*; and Laudan, *Cuisine and Empire*, 297–98.

19 Shelley, *The Complete Poetical Works of Shelley*, 609; "Guide to London," 1893–1894; and "Letter to the *Natal Mercury*," February 3, 1896.

20 Gandhi, "Ahimsa and Other Animals"; Hay, "The Making of a Late-Victorian Hindu," 89–90; and Hunt, *Gandhi in London*, 221.

21 Kingsford, *The Perfect Way in Diet*, 19; Stuart, *The Bloodless Revolution*; "Letter to Mrs. A. M. Lewis," August 4, 1894; "Books for Sale," *Natal Mercury*, November 28, 1894; "Letter to R. B. Gregg," May 27, 1927; Hill, "The Vegetarian Federal Union"; and "The Vegetarian Federal Union," *Vegetarian (London)*, October 12, 1889.

22 "Letter to Henry S. Salt," October 28, 1932; "Speech at Meeting of London Vegetarian Society," November 20, 1931; and Lelyveld, *Great Soul*, 83.

23 "The Deputation's Voyage—VI," *Indian Opinion*, December 1, 1906; and "To the Editor," *Natal Mercury*, February 4, 1896.

24 "Vegetarianism in Natal," *Vegetarian*, December 21, 1895; "To the Editor," *Natal Mercury*, February 2, 1896; and King, *The Papers of Martin Luther King, Jr.*, 119.

25 "To the Editor," *Natal Mercury*, February 4, 1896; and *Natal Advertiser*, February 1, 1895.

26 Corman, "The Ventriloquist's Burden."

27 "Letter to R. B. Gregg," May 27, 1927; Hills, "The Vegetarian Federal Union"; "The Vegetarian Federal Union," *Vegetarian*, October 12, 1889; "Portsmouth Mission," *Vegetarian*, May 9, 1891; and "The Federal Union Report," *Vegetarian*, May 23, 1891.

28 "The Foods of India," *Vegetarian Messenger*, June 1, 1891.

29 Gandhi, *An Autobiography*, 50–53.

30 Gandhi, *An Autobiography*, 51–52.

31 "Speech to the Band of Mercy, London," *Vegetarian*, June 6, 1891; and "Speech at Farewell Dinner," *Vegetarian*, June 11, 1891.

32 Albert West, "In the Early Days with Gandhi—I"; and Guha, *Gandhi before India*, 165.

33 Gandhi, *An Autobiography*, 133–34.

34 "Vegetarianism in Natal," *Vegetarian*, December 21, 1895; "To the Editor," *Natal Mercury*, February 4, 1896.

35 Shprintzen, *The Vegetarian Crusade*, 2.

36 "My Notes," *Navajivan*, December 11, 1921.

37 "Vegetarianism in Natal," *Vegetarian*, December 21, 1895; and "Letter to the *Vegetarian*," April 28, 1894.

38 Ray, *The Migrant's Table*, 44; Bryant, "Strategies of Vedic Subversion"; "Guide to London," 1893 or 1894; "Letter to V. G. Desai," May 14, 1924; and "Letter to Akbarbhai Chavda," December 2, 1944.

39 Salt, *The Logic of Vegetarianism*, 10; "Indian Vegetarians—I," *Vegetarian*, February 7, 1891; and "The Foods of India," *Vegetarian Messenger*, June 1, 1891.

40 Scrinis, *Nutritionism*, 47; Djousse and Gaziano, "Egg Consumption"; "Deputation's Voyage [II]," before July 9, 1909; "Letter to Jamnadas Gandhi," March 29, 1913; "A Letter," before July 7, 1927; "Letter to Narandas Gandhi," October 16, 1930; and "Letter to Bal Kalelkar," February 12, 1933.

41 "Discussion with B. G. Kher and Others," August 15, 1940.

42 Desai, *Diary of Mahadev Desai*, 21.

43 Safi, "Muslim Man Dies in India in India after Attack by Hindu 'Cow Protectors'"; Dosanjh, "Cow Vigilantism Threatens the Body and Soul of India"; and Laudan, *Cuisine and Empire*, 298.

44 Gandhi, *Hind Swaraj*, 46–47; "Speech at Gujarati Political Conference—I," November 3, 1917; and *Young India*, October 6, 1921.

45 "Hindu-Muslim Unity," *Navajivan*, February 29, 1920.

46 "Letter to Asaf Ali," January 25, 1920.

47 "Let Hindus Beware," *Young India*, May 18, 1921; and "Advice to People of Gaya," May 29, 1921.

48 "Discussion on Boycott at AICC Meeting," *Navajivan*, September 11, 1921.

49 Tolstoy, *The Kingdom of God Is Within You*; Murthy, *Mahatma Gandhi and Leo Tolstoy Letters*; Lavrin, "Tolstoy and Gandhi"; Tolstoy, "The First Step," 97–106; Wilson, *Tolstoy*; Bartlett, *Tolstoy*; and "Leo Tolstoi," *Vegetarian*, December 21, 1889.

50 "Letter to Ranchhodlal Patwari," June 10, 1915; *Young India*, October 6, 1921; "Letter to Narahari Parikh," February 13, 1920; "Speech at Meeting of London Vegetarian Society," November 20, 1931; and "Speech at Meeting of London Vegetarian Society," November 20, 1931.

51 Quoted in Weber, *On the Salt March*, 429.

52 Smith-Howard, *Pure and Modern Milk*, 11; Valenze, *Milk*; Wiley, "Milk for 'Growth'"; Dupuis, *Nature's Perfect Food*; Mahias, "Milk and Its Transmutations in Indian Society"; and "Food," in *Key to Health*, December 18, 1942.

53 Weber, *Gandhi as Disciple and Mentor*, 35; Sharma, *Gandhi*, 43–45; Roy, *Alimentary Tracts*, 112; and "Raw v. Cooked Food," *Navajivan*, June 16, 1929.

54 "Letter to Maganlal Gandhi," October 25, 1914; and "Letter to Maganlal Gandhi," December 10, 1914.

55 Gandhi, *An Autobiography*, 298–99.

56 "Letter to Ranchhodlal Patwari," June 10, 1915; "Letter to Maganbhai H. Patel," December 12, 1915; Polak, *Mr. Gandhi*, 70–87; and Guha, *Gandhi before India*, 199–200.

57 In a letter Gandhi wrote in 1919, as well as in his autobiography, he attributed the idea of goat's milk to Kasturba. In *Key to Health*, it is the doctor that suggests goat's milk and Kasturba who seconds the idea. See "Letter to Maganlal Gandhi," January 10, 1919; Gandhi, *An Autobiography*, 227–28 and 378; and "Food," in *Key to Health*, December 18, 1942.

58 "Food," in *Key to Health*, December 18, 1942; "Letter to Haribhau Upadhyaya," July 12, 1929; "General Knowledge about Health [XIII]," *Indian Opinion*, March 29, 1913; "Letter to Bhaishir Chhaganlal," December 10, 1928; "Letter to Rameshchandra," December 13, 1927; "Letter to Mahadev Desai," November 30, 1928; "Letter to Richard B. Gregg," January 28, 1929; "Some Questions," *Navajivan*, September 27, 1925; and "Letter to a Friend," August 9, 1918.

59 "General Knowledge about Health [XII]," *Indian Opinion*, March 22, 1913; "Letter to a Friend," August 9, 1918; and "Food," in *Key to Health*, December 18, 1942.

60 "Food," in *Key to Health*, December 18, 1942; "Letter to P. C. Ray," August 27, 1918; and "General Knowledge about Health [XIII]," *Indian Opinion*, March 29, 1913.

61 "Letter to Hermann Kallenbach," October 23, 1915; and "The Foods of India," *Vegetarian Messenger*, June 1, 1891.

62 "General Knowledge about Health [XIII]," *Indian Opinion*, March 29, 1913; "Letter to Haribhau Upadhyaya," July 12, 1929; and "Letter to Narandas Gandhi," January 1/6, 1931.

63 Slate, *Colored Cosmopolitanism*, 101–7; "Letter to P. C. Ray," August 27, 1918; and Mazumdar, "The Impact of New World Food Crops on the Diet and Economy of China and India."

64 "Letter to D. Hanumantrao," April 5, 1924; and "Letter to C. F. Andrews," August 13, 1921.

65 "Some Questions," *Navajivan*, September 27, 1925; "Letter to a Friend," August 9, 1918; "Speech at Gujarati Political Conference," November 3, 1917; "Speech at Women's Meeting, Dakor," *Navajivan*, November 3, 1920; "Child

Mortality," *Navajivan*, January 11, 1920; "Letter to Devdas Gandhi," November 1920; "Food," in *Key to Health*, December 18, 1942; and "Speech at Prayer Meeting," May 1, 1947.

66 "Food," in *Key to Health*, December 18, 1942; "Rejoinder," *Young India*, December 15, 1920; "On Trial," *Young India*, November 20, 1924; "A Taxing Examiner," *Young India*, April 6, 1921; "Talk to Students at Dacca," May 17, 1925; "Letter to Syed Zahirul Haq," November 10, 1926; and "Speech at Education Ministers' Conference," July 29, 1946.

67 "Speech at Prayer Meeting," June 29, 1947.

68 "Unfired Food," *Young India*, August 15, 1929.

69 Merton, "Gandhi and the One-Eyed Giant," 7 and 10. Italics in original.

70 "Letter to G. D. Birla," after March 11, 1924; Brown, *Gandhi's Rise to Power*, 42; and Guha, *Gandhi before India*, 545.

CHAPTER 4: RAW, WHOLE, REAL

Epigraph: "Letter to Maganlal Gandhi," November 27, 1909.

1 "Work for Vegetarianism," *Vegetarian*, April 16, 1892.

2 "An Experiment in Vital Food," March 24, *Vegetarian*, 1894.

3 "An Experiment in Vital Food," March 24, *Vegetarian*, 1894; "Letter to Haribhau Upadhyaya," July 12, 1929; "General Knowledge about Health [XII]," *Indian Opinion*, March 22, 1913; "Raw v. Cooked Food," *Navajivan*, June 16, 1929; "Green Leaves," *Harijan*, February 15, 1935; "Ashram Notes," February 7, 1942; and "Unfired Food Experiment," *Young India*, July 18, 1929.

4 Lévi-Strauss, *The Raw and the Cooked*; Johnson and Boswell, *A Journey to the Western Islands of Scotland*, 172; and Wrangham, *Catching Fire*.

5 "General Knowledge about Health [XIII]," *Indian Opinion*, March 29, 1913; "Letter to V. S. Srinivasa Sastri," May 14, 1915; and "Letter to Chhaganlal Gandhi," December 23, 1914.

6 "Letter to Hermann Kallenbach," March 15, 1914.

7 Gandhi, *An Autobiography*, 298–99; and Allinson, *Dr. Allinson's Cookery Book*.

8 Guha, *Gandhi before India*, 360.

9 "The Foods of India," *Vegetarian Messenger*, June 1, 1891.

10 "Green Leaves," *Harijan*, February 15, 1935; "Ashram Notes," February 7, 1942; and "Letter to Maganlal Gandhi," December 10, 1914.

11 "Raw v. Cooked Food," *Navajivan*, June 16, 1929.

12 Ibid.

13 "Raw v. Cooked Food," *Navajivan*, June 16, 1929; "Unfired Food Experiment," *Young India*, July 18, 1929; Desai, *Diary of Mahadev Desai*, 26; "Letter to Harilal Gandhi," September 9, 1918; "Food," in *Key to Health*, December 18, 1942; Petrini, *Slow Food*; and Andrews, *The Slow Food Story*.

14 "General Knowledge about Health [XI]," *Indian Opinion*, March 15, 1913.

15 Shapiro, *Perfection Salad*; "To the All India Women's Conference," 1936; and Kishwar, "Gandhi on Women," 1691.

16 "Letter to Mirabehn," February 2, 1933.

17 "Unfired Food Experiment," *Young India*, July 18, 1929.

18 Larson, Story, and Nelson, "Neighborhood Environments"; Amsden and Amsden, *The Rawvolution Continues*; and Kenney, *Cooked Raw*.

19 "Unfired Food Experiment," *Young India*, July 18, 1929.

20 "Letter to Rani Vidyavati," July 15, 1929; "Letter to Vallabhbhai Patel," February 7, 1942; and "Letter to Hermann Kallenbach," July 10, 1914.

21 Levenstein, *Revolution at the Table*, 89–92.

22 "Ashram Notes," February 7, 1942.

23 "Civilization or Barbarism?" after September 18, 1909.

24 Mintz, *Tasting Food, Tasting Freedom*, 84–91; and Douglas, *Purity and Danger*.

25 Sharma, "Food and Empire," 242; Maroney, "'To Make a Curry the India Way'"; Zlotnick, "Domesticating Imperialism"; Leong-Salobir, *Food Culture in Colonial Asia*, chapter 2; Collingham, *Curry*, 251; and Burton, *The Raj at Table*.

26 "Mistaken Humanity," *Young India*, October 4, 1928.

27 "Letter to Chhaganlal Gandhi," May 1, 1905; "Letter to Haji Ismail Haji Aboobaker Johari," August 14, 1906; "Letter to Dr. Pranjivan Mehta," August 7, 1911; and Gandhi, *Hind Swaraj*, 33.

28 Cort, *Jains in the World*, 118–41; Laidlaw, *Riches and Renunciation*; *Indian Opinion*, August 16, 1913; "Diary for 1915," April 9, 1915; "Letter to H. Kallenbach," August 10, 1920; "Letter to Amtussalaam," January 2, 1934; "Letter to Chhaganlal Joshi," February 9, 1934; and "Letter to Maganlal Gandhi," about 1914.

29 "Letter to Narandas Gandhi," May 4, 1915.

30 "Letter to Jamnadas Gandhi," March 22, 1914.

31 "Letter to Mirabehn," February 2, 1933; and "Letter to Premabehn Kantak," March 6, 1933. Also see Pollan, *Cooked*: 339–41.

32 "Letter to Maganlal Gandhi," December 10, 1914.

33 "Letter to Maganlal Gandhi," about 1914.

34 "Letter to Mahadev Desai," May 9, 1918; and "Letter to Chhaganlal Gandhi," April 24, 1912.

35 "Letter to Maganlal Gandhi," about 1914; and Meyer-Renschausen, "The Porridge Debate."

36 Graham, *Treatise on Bread and Bread-Making*, preface; and Lobel, "Sylvester Graham and Antebellum Diet Reform."

37 Pollan, *Cooked*, 256–61.

38 Allinson's name still graces a popular brand of bread. See "Letter to Hermann Kallenbach," December 26, 1914; and Allinson, *The Advantages of Wholemeal Bread*.

39 "Letter to R. B. Gregg," May 27, 1927; Anonymous, "Bread Reform League"; Forward, *Fifty Years of Food Reform*, 82–83; and Anonymous, "The Leader of the W.W.C.T.U. Food Reform Movement."

40 "Indian Vegetarians III," *Vegetarian*, February 21, 1891; "The Foods of India," *Vegetarian Messenger*, June 1, 1891; "Food" in *Key to Health*, December 18, 1942; "Unfired Food Experiment," *Young India*, July 18, 1929; and "General Knowledge about Health [XII]," *Indian Opinion*, March 22, 1913.

41 "Letter to R. B. Gregg," May 27, 1927.

42 Kipling, "William the Conqueror—Part II"; McCarrison, "A Good Diet and a Bad One"; McCarrison, "Problems of Nutrition in India," 267–68; Vernon, *Hunger*, 106; Laudan, *Cuisine and Empire*, 269; McCay, *The Protein Element in Nutrition*, 51 and 178; Streets, *Martial Races*; and Sinha, *Colonial Masculinity*.

43 "Food" in *Key to Health*, December 18, 1942; "Letter to Haribhau Phatak," January 29, 1935; "Indian Vegetarians III," *Vegetarian*, February 21, 1891; "The Foods of India," *Vegetarian Messenger*, June 1, 1891; "Evils of Machine-Milling," *Young India*, May 12, 1927; and Carpenter, *Beriberi, White Rice, and Vitamin B*.

44 "Food" in *Key to Health*, December 18, 1942; "Letter to Haribhau Phatak," January 29, 1935; "Letter to Sumangal Prakash," March 20, 1933; and "Letter to Narandas Gandhi," November 6, 1932.

45 "Food" in *Key to Health*, December 18, 1942; "General Knowledge about Health [XXIII]," *Indian Opinion*, June 7, 1913; and "General Knowledge about Health [XXVIII]," *Indian Opinion*, July 12, 1913.

46 "Some Questions," *Navajivan*, September 27, 1925.

47 "Letter to Mirabehn," November 3, 1932.

48 "Letter to G. D. Birla," after March 11, 1924; "Letter to Ramdas Gandhi," June 1, 1919; and "General Knowledge about Health [XI]," *Indian Opinion*, March 15, 1913.

49 "General Knowledge about Health [XI]," *Indian Opinion*, March 15, 1913; "Food" in *Key to Health*, December 18, 1942; and "Letter to V. S. Srinivasa Sastri," May 14, 1915.

50 "General Knowledge about Health [XI]," *Indian Opinion*, March 15, 1913.

51 "The Last Satyagraha Campaign: Preface," *Indian Opinion*, August 26, 1914; "Letter to Hermann Kallenbach," March 2, 1915; "Letter to Hermann Kallenbach," August 1, 1913; "Letter to Hermann Kallenbach," January 28, 1915; and "Letter to Hermann Kallenbach," March 9, 1914.

52 "Letter to Devdas Gandhi," November, 1920; "General Knowledge about Health [XIII]," *Indian Opinion*, March 29, 1913; and "Letter to Hermann Kallenbach," March 31, 1913.

53 "Letter to Jamnadas Gandhi," March 17, 1914; and "Letter to Hermann Kallenbach," March 21, 1915.

54 "Letter to Jamnadas Gandhi," March 17, 1914.

55 "Letter to Jamnadas Gandhi," March 17, 1914. Also see Cort, *Jains in the World*, 129.

56 "Letter to Jamnadas Gandhi," March 17, 1914.

57 "Letter to Narandas Gandhi," November 6, 1932.

58 "Green Leaves," *Harijan*, February 15, 1935; "Letter to Kanti Gandhi," November 9, 1934; "Ashram Notes," February 7, 1942; Alport, *Queen of Fats*; and Doctor, "Purslane."

59 "Green Leaves," *Harijan*, February 15, 1935; Berson, "The Quinoa Conundrum"; and Hamilton, "The Quinoa Quarrel."

60 Hayes et al., "The Cancer Chemopreventive Actions of Phytochemicals"; Murillo and Mehta, "Cruciferous Vegetables and Cancer Prevention"; Kivelä et al., "Sulforaphane Inhibits Endothelial Lipase Expression"; and Yao, "Flavonoids in Food and Their Health Benefits."

61 "Green Leaves," *Harijan*, February 15, 1935; Freidberg, *Fresh*; Nestle, "Paleolithic Diets"; Cordain, *The Paleo Diet*; and Cordain et al., "Origins and Evolution of the Western Diet."

62 Gandhi, *Hind Swaraj*, 53–54.

CHAPTER 5: NATURAL MEDICINE

Epigraph: "General Knowledge about Health I," *Indian Opinion*, January 4, 1913.

1 Arnold, *Gandhi*, 225–27; Nandy, "Final Encounter"; "Notes," *Young India*, June 1, 1921; and Shetty, "The Quack Whom We Know."

2 "Speech at Prayer Meeting," December 29, 1947; and Digby et al., *Crossing Colonial Historiographies*.

3 "General Knowledge about Health I," *Indian Opinion*, January 4, 1913; and Svoboda, *Ayurveda*, 112.

4 "Speech at Ashtanga Ayurveda Vidyalala," *Amrita Bazar Patrika*, May 8, 1925.

5 "Ayurveda and Nature Cure," *Harijan*, May 19, 1946.

6 "Letter to Vasumati D. Pandit," January 18, 1945; and Stacey, *Consumed*, 213.

7 Apple, *Vitamania*; Willett, *Eat, Drink, and Be Healthy*; and Lichtenstein and Russell, "Essential Nutrients."

8 "Letter to 'Prajabandhu,'" April 20, 1916; "Letter to D. B. Kalelkar," August 4, 1926; and "Letter to R. B. Gregg," April 26, 1927.

9 "Letter to R. B. Gregg," May 13, 1927; "Letter to R. B. Gregg," May 27, 1927; Kosek, "Richard Gregg, Mohandas Gandhi, and the Strategy of Nonviolence";

"Letter to Dr. M. S. Kelkar," May 28, 1927; and Plimmer and Plimmer, *Food, Health, Vitamins.*

10 "Letter to Satis Chandra Das Gupta," May 12, 1928; "My Notes," *Navajivan,* September, 9, 1928; "Raw v. Cooked Food," *Navajivan,* June 16, 1929; and "Mistaken Humanity," *Young India,* October 4, 1928.

11 "Unfired Food," *Young India,* August 15, 1929.

12 Harrison, *Climates and Constitutions*; and Collingham, *Imperial Bodies,* 90.

13 "Letter to Tarabehn R. Modi," March 8, 1934; and Alter, *Gandhi's Body,* chapter 3.

14 Gandhi, *Hind Swaraj,* 53–54; Kaufman, *Homeopathy in America*; and Haller, *The History of Homeopathy.*

15 "Speech at Ashtanga Ayurveda Vidyalala," *Amrita Bazar Patrika,* May 8, 1925; and "Discussion with Dr. Chesterman," February 13, 1939.

16 "Speech at Ashtanga Ayurveda Vidyalala," *Amrita Bazar Patrika,* May 8, 1925; and "Letter to Vallabhram Vaidya," June 28, 1942.

17 "Speech at Gondal Rasashala," January 27, 1915; and "Letter to Gangadhar Shastri Joshi," July 19, 1927.

18 Langford, *Fluent Bodies,* 108.

19 "Speech at Ashtanga Ayurveda Vidyalala," *Amrita Bazar Patrika,* May 8, 1925.

20 "Ayurvedic System," *Young India,* June 11, 1925; and "Letter to Vallabhram Vaidya," June 28, 1942.

21 "Letter to Gangadhar Shastri Joshi," July 19, 1927; "Letter to Shiv Sharma," November 30, 1944; "Letter to Mathuradas Trikumji," January 1, 1945; "Letter to Shiv Sharma," January 18, 1945; "Letter to C. Rajagopalachari," January 1, 1945; "Letter to Vallabhram Vaidya," December 4, 1945; and "Letter to Vallabhram Vaidya," June 8, 1942.

22 "Ayurvedic System," *Young India,* June 11, 1925.

23 "Speech at Prayer Meeting," November 1, 1947.

24 "Letter to Gokhale," December 4, 1912.

25 "Letter to V. S. Srinivasa Sastri," November 5, 1918; and "Discussion with Dr. Chesterman," February 13, 1939.

26 "Water," in *Key to Health,* December 18, 1942.

27 "Letter to Akbarbhai Chavda," December 2, 1944; "Letter to Vasumati D. Pandit," January 18, 1945; "Neem Leaves and Tamarind," *Harijan,* November 16, 1935; and "Letter to R. B. Gregg," April 26, 1927. Also see "Neem" on WebMD, www.webmd.com/vitamins/ai/ingredientmono-577/neem.

28 Aykroyd, "Beriberi and Other Food-Deficiency Diseases"; Aykroyd, "Nutrition and Public Health"; Carpenter, "The Work of Wallace Aykroyd"; and "Neem Leaves and Tamarind," *Harijan,* November 16, 1935.

29 "An Aspiring Naturopath," *Harijan,* December 14, 1934.

30 "Neem Leaves and Tamarind," *Harijan*, November 16, 1935; and "Speech to Village Workers," *Harijan*, November 2, 1935.

31 "Neem Leaves and Tamarind," *Harijan*, November 16, 1935; and "Letter to S. Ambujammal," October 15, 1935.

32 "Note to Krishnachandra," March 7, 1945; "Letter to Bachubhai D. Ramdas," March 10, 1936; "Letter to Tara N. Mashruwala," March 21, 1936; "Letter to Prabhavati," June 30, 1936; and "Letter to Subhas Chandra Bose," September 13, 1936.

33 "Soya Beans," *Harijan*, November 9, 1935.

34 "Letter to Vasumati D. Pandit," January 18, 1945; and "Letter to Subhas Chandra Bose," September 13, 1936.

35 Katz, *The Selected Papers of Margaret Sanger*, entry 106; "Letter to Budhabhai," November 9, 1930.

36 "Letter to Mirabehn," August 26, 1941; "Guide to London," 1893–94; and "Letter to Chandan Parekh," May 24, 1939.

37 "Letter to Anand T. Hingorani," January 9, 1945; "Ayurveda and Nature Cure," *Harijan*, May 19, 1946; "Letter to Jamnalal Bajaj," March 16, 1939; "Letter to Madalasa," October 15, 1941; "On Brahmacharya," *Harijanbandhu*, October 22, 1939; and "Ayurvedic System," *Young India*, June 11, 1925.

38 "Letter to Gangadhar Shastri Joshi," July 19, 1927.

39 Gandhi, *An Autobiography*, 205–7.

40 "Letter to Akbarbhai Chavda," December 2, 1944; "Ayurveda and Nature Cure," *Harijan*, May 19, 1946; and "General Knowledge about Health, III," *Indian Opinion*, January 18, 1913.

41 "Letter to Akbarbhai Chavda," December 2, 1944; "Ayurveda and Nature Cure," *Harijan*, May 19, 1946; and "General Knowledge about Health, III," *Indian Opinion*, January 18, 1913.

42 "Speech to Village Workers," *Harijan*, November 2, 1935.

43 "Letter to Chhaganlal Gandhi," April 19, 1917; and "Letter to Hermann Kallenbach," April 1, 1916.

CHAPTER 6: FARMING

Epigraph: "To Shambhushanker," August 30, 1926.

1 "Speech at Bhagini Samaj, Bombay," October 2, 1919; and Berry, *What Are People For?*, 145.

2 "Rural Education," *Shikshan ane Sahitya*, August 18, 1929; "Implications of Constructive Programme," *Harijan*, August 18, 1940; Maine, *Village-Communities in the East and West*; and Mantena, *Alibis of Empire*.

3 Gandhi, *An Autobiography*, 248–49; "Sarvodaya," *Indian Opinion*, May 16, 1908.

4 Kaufman, *Bet the Farm*; Hesterman, *Fair Food*; and Winne, *Closing the Food Gap*.

5 "A Primer 3," April 14, 1922.

6 "A Primer 3," April 14, 1922.

7 "Work for Vegetarianism," *Vegetarian*, September 20, 1893.

8 "General Knowledge about Health [XV]," *Indian Opinion*, April 12, 1913; "Letter to Budhabhai," November 9, 1930; "Letter to Chhaganlal Gandhi," May 6, 1905; and "Tyranny of Law," *Indian Opinion*, June 15, 1907.

9 "Letter to Narandas Gandhi," September 14/16, 1930; and "Letter to Narandas Gandhi," May 1/2, 1933.

10 "Letter to Narandas Gandhi," May 1/2, 1933.

11 "Letter to Chanchalbehn Gandhi," February 26, 1909; and "Letter to Maganlal Gandhi," December 10, 1914.

12 "General Knowledge about Health [XV]," *Indian Opinion*, April 12, 1913.

13 "Unfired Food," *Young India*, August 15, 1929.

14 "Supreme Virtue of Agriculture," *Indian Opinion*, December 3, 1910.

15 Ibid.

16 "Food," in *Key to Health*, December 18, 1942.

17 Robidoux and Mason, *A Land Not Forgotten*; Naylor, *The Evolving Sphere of Food Security*; and Brown, *Full Planet, Empty Plates*.

18 "Speech to Village Workers," *Harijan*, November 2, 1935; Sholten, *India's White Revolution*; and Shanti, *Operation Flood*.

19 "Food," in *Key to Health*, December 18, 1942.

20 *Natal Mercury*, February 4, 1897; "The Indian Famine," July 30, 1900; and Vernon, *Hunger*, 69.

21 *Natal Mercury*, February 4, 1897; and "The Indian Famine," July 30, 1900.

22 "Appeal for Funds," *Natal Advertiser*, February 4, 1897.

23 "Home Rule for India," *Indian Opinion*, May 12, 1906; Sen, *Poverty and Famines*; and Davis, *Late Victorian Holocausts*.

24 "The Great Sentinel," *Young India*, October 13, 1921.

25 "Discussion at Food Conference," November 6, 1947; "Silence Day Note to R. G. Casey," December 3, 1945; "Statement to the United Press of India," February 7, 1946; "Letter to R. G. Casey," February 8, 1946; Mukerjee, *Churchill's Secret War*; and Aykroyd, *The Conquest of Famine*.

26 "Letter to R. G. Casey," December 8, 1945.

27 "Vegetarianism in Natal," *Vegetarian*, December 21, 1895.

28 Marable, *African Nationalist*; Davis, "John L. Dube"; Hunt, "Gandhi and the Black People of South Africa"; and "Negroes Welcome Rev. Andrews, Missionary from India," *Daily Chronicle*, June 17, 1929, I/D 231, Benarsidas Chaturvedi Papers, National Archives of India.

29 "From Slave to College President," *Indian Opinion*, October 9, 1903; Guha, *Gandhi before India*, 175; and Hofmeyer, *Gandhi's Printing Press*.

30 "Count Tolstoy," *Indian Opinion*, September 2, 1905.

31 "Count Tolstoy," *Indian Opinion*, September 2, 1905; "Count Tolstoi and his Work," *Vegetarian*, January 23, 1890.

32 "Gandhi to Tolstoy," October 1, 1909, in Murthy, *Mahatma Gandhi and Leo Tolstoy Letters*.

33 "Tolstoy to Gandhi," Oct. 7, 1909, in Murthy, *Mahatma Gandhi and Leo Tolstoy Letters*.

34 "Gandhi to Tolstoy," November 10, 1909, "Gandhi to Tolstoy," April 4, 1910, "Tolstoy to Gandhi," May 8, 1910, "Gandhi to Tolstoy," Aug 15, 1910, and "Tolstoy to Gandhi," September 7, 1910, all in Murthy, *Mahatma Gandhi and Leo Tolstoy Letters*; and McKeogh, *Tolstoy's Pacifism*, 122.

35 "Tolstoy to Gandhi," September 7, 1910, in Murthy, *Mahatma Gandhi and Leo Tolstoy Letters*; and "Preface to Leo Tolstoy's 'Letter to a Hindoo,'" November 19, 1909.

36 Gandhi, *Satyagraha in South Africa*, 221–22.

37 Ibid.

38 "Satyagrahi Farm," *Indian Opinion*, June 25, 1910.

39 Ibid.

40 "Trading Licenses in the Transvaal," *Indian Opinion*, October 22, 1910; and "Satyagrahi Farm," *Indian Opinion*, June 25, 1910.

41 Slate, *Colored Cosmopolitanism*, 24–25; and Lelyveld, *Great Soul*, 93.

42 "Tolstoy Farm," *Indian Opinion*, June 18, 1910.

43 "Transvaal Notes," *Indian Opinion*, January 21, 1911; "Satyagrahi Farm," *Indian Opinion*, July 9, 1910; and "Letter to Maganlal Gandhi," December 10, 1914.

44 Drayton, *Nature's Government*.

45 "Letter to Sir Robert McCarrison," November 5, 1934; "AIFIA—Object and Constitution," December 14, 1934; Conford, *The Origins of the Organic Movement*; McCarrison, "Nutrition in Health and Disease"; McCarrison, "The Relation of Manure"; and Lockeretz, *Organic Farming*, 11, 25, 47, 61.

46 Warboys, "The Discovery of Colonial Malnutrition between the Wars"; Arnold, "The 'Discovery' of Malnutrition and Diet in Colonial India"; Arnold, *Colonizing the Body*; and Hauter, *Foodopoly*, 3.

47 Prasad, *Satyagraha in Champaran*, 201.

48 "The Foods of India," *Vegetarian Messenger*, June 1, 1891; and "Letter to R. B. Gregg," May 29, 1927.

49 Guha, *Dominance without Hegemony*, 37–38; Das Gupta, *Gandhi's Economic Thought*; and Dutt, "Rajani Palme Dutt," 403.

50 Guha, *India after Gandhi*, 226–27; and Herring, *Land to the Tiller*.

51 "The Pyramid vs. the Oceanic Circle," 1946.

52 Mehta, *Mahatma Gandhi and His Apostles*, 4–5.

53 "Speech at Subjects Committee Meeting, AICC," October 24, 1934.

Epigraph: "A Note," August 1947.

1 Tolstoy, "The First Step," 97; Pearson, *Because It Gives Me Peace of Mind*; Bynum, *Holy Feast and Holy Fast*.

2 Mintz, *Tasting Food, Tasting Freedom*, 4; Laidlaw, "A Life Worth Leaving"; Arnold, *Decoding Anorexia*; and Brumberg, *Fasting Girls*.

3 "A Note," August 1947.

4 "Letter to Dr. Pranjivan Mehta," August 7, 1911; and Mehta, *Mahatma Gandhi and His Apostles*, 48.

5 "The Physical Effects of Fasting," *Young India*, December 17, 1925.

6 "The Physical Effects of Fasting," *Young India*, December 17, 1925; and "Letter to Hermann Kallenbach," on or before April 3, 1911.

7 "The Physical Effects of Fasting," *Young India*, December 17, 1925; "Letter to Hermann Kallenbach," July 24, 1913; and "Letter to Narahari Parikh," February 21, 1924.

8 "General Knowledge about Health, IX," *Indian Opinion*, March 1, 1913; "Letter to Budhabhai," November 9, 1930; and "Guide to London," 1893-94.

9 "The Physical Effects of Fasting," *Young India*, December 17, 1925; "Letter to Dr. N. R. Dharmavir," September 5, 1934; and "Notes," *Harijan*, August 24, 1934.

10 "The Physical Effects of Fasting," *Young India*, December 17, 1925.

11 Butterly and Shepherd, *Hunger*; and Hendricks, "Starving Your Way to Vigor."

12 "Appeal to Bombay Citizens," November 19, 1921; and "The Physical Effects of Fasting," *Young India*, December 17, 1925.

13 Gandhi, *An Autobiography*, 4.

14 "Letter to H. S. L. Polak," October 26, 1906; "General Knowledge about Health, XIV," *Indian Opinion*, April 5, 1913; "England and Russia," *Indian Opinion*, November 26, 1903; "Letter to Private Secretary to Lore Crewe," September 18, 1909; and "Letter to the Press," October 10, 1919.

15 "General Knowledge about Health, XI," Indian Opinion, April 5, 1913; and "The Physical Effects of Fasting," *Young India*, December 17, 1925.

16 "The Physical Effects of Fasting," *Young India*, December 17, 1925; and "Some Questions," *Navajivan*, September 27, 1925.

17 "Id Greetings," *Indian Opinion*, November 9, 1907; and "Letter to Maganlal Gandhi," August 31, 1910.

18 "Fasting and Prayer," *Navajivan*, October 12, 1919; "Letter to V. S. Srinivasa Sastri," March 20, 1920; and "Letter to Hermann Kallenbach," July 24, 1913, July 25, 1913, July 30, 1913, and August 18, 1913.

19 "Satyagraha Leaflet No. 17," May 7, 1919.

20 "Letter to V. S. Srinivasa Sastri," March 20, 1920.

21 "Satyagraha Leaflet No. 15," May 5, 1919.

22 "Suffragettes," *Indian Opinion*, August 28, 1909; Vernon, *Hunger*, 60–80; and Grant, "British Suffragettes and the Russian Method of Hunger Strike."

23 Gandhi, *An Autobiography*, 285-287; and Guha, *Gandhi before India*, 458–60.

24 "Letter to the Press," May 26, 1909; "Letter to Hermann Kallenbach," September 23, 1911; "Letter to Hermann Kallenbach," October 14, 1911; "Letter to Harilal Gandhi," September 5, 1912; "Letter to Maganlal Gandhi," November 11, 1913; "Speech at Mass Meeting," December 21, 1913; and "Letter to Manibehn Patel," April 27, 1945.

25 "Letter to Manilal Gandhi," April 17, 1914; "Speech on 'Ashram Vows' at YMCA, Madras," February 16, 1916; "Speech at Muir College Economic Society, Allahabad," December 22, 1916; "Speech at Women's Meeting, Bombay," May 8, 1919; "Village Industries," *Harijan*, November 16, 1934; "Speech at Students' Meeting, Banaras," November 26, 1920; and "Speech at Merchants' Meeting, Calcutta," January 26, 1921.

26 "My Loin-Cloth," *Navajivan*, July 27, 1924.

27 "Statement to the Press," December 1, 1944.

28 "Letter to the Press," *Leader*, April 3, 1918; "Ahmedabad Mill-Hands' Strike," March 16, 1918; and Suhrud, "Emptied of All but Love."

29 "Speech to Ahmedabad Mill-Hands," March 15, 1918; "Letter to the Press," *Leader*, April 3, 1918; "Letter to Devdas Gandhi," April 12, 1918; and "Letter to Esther Faering," April 8, 1918.

30 "Prayer Discourse in Ashram," March 17, 1918; "Letter to the Press," *Leader*, April 3, 1918; and "Letter to Esther Faering," April 8, 1918.

31 "Fragment of Letter to Ambalal Sarabhai," March 17, 1918; and "Address to Ashram Inmates," March 18, 1918.

32 "Some Questions," *Navajivan*, September 27, 1925.

33 "Gandhi Diary," 1915; and "Letter to Hermann Kallenbach," October 23, 1915.

34 "Notes," *Young India*, December 8, 1921.

35 "Letter to a Friend," February 2, 1921.

36 "Satyagraha Leaflet no. 17," May 7, 1919.

37 "Letter to George Joseph," April 12, 1924; "Notes," *Young India*, July 31, 1924; and "Vaikom Satyagraha," *Young India*, May 1, 1924.

38 King, *Gandhian Nonviolent Struggle*.

39 For Gandhi's views on caste, see Arnold, *Gandhi*, 169–74; and Nagaraj, *The Flaming Feet and Other Essays*.

40 Zelliot, *Ambedkar's World*; and Jaffrelot, *Dr. Ambedkar and Untouchability*.

41 "Telegram to Secretary, Home Department," April 30, 1933.

42 Ambedkar, *What Congress and Gandhi Have Done to the Untouchables*, 286–88, 298–99; "Caste 'versus' Class," *Young India*, December 29, 1920; and "A Catechism," *Young India*, October 14, 1926.

43 "Caste Has to Go," *Harijan*, November 16, 1935; "Question Box," *Harijan*, June 15, 1940; and Kumar, *Radical Equality*.

44 "Statement Announcing Twenty-One-Day Fast," September 18, 1924.

45 "Discussion with C. Rajagopalachari," September 1, 1947.

46 "Letter to Vallabhbhai Patel," September 1, 1947.

47 "Statement to the Press," September 1, 1947; "Letter to Vallabhbhai Patel," September 1/2, 1947; "Discussion with Hindu-Muslim Representatives," September 3, 1947; and "Discussion with a Deputation," September 4, 1947.

48 Dalton, *Mahatma Gandhi*, 155–56.

49 "Advice to Demonstrators," September 4, 1947.

50 "Discussion With A Deputation," September 4, 1947.

51 "Speech before Breaking of Fast," September 4, 1947.

CONCLUSION: MANGOES AND MAHATMAS

Epigraph: "Letter to Sarladevi Chowdhrani," May 1, 1920.

1 "Note to Amrita Lal Chatterjee," April 15, 1941.

2 Shenker, "E. B. White."

3 "Punjab Letter," November 25, 1919; Gandhi, *Mohandas*, 229–34; Green, *Gandhi*, 223–26 and 273–85; and Ray, *Early Feminists of Colonial India*.

4 "Letter to Saraladevi Chowdharani," December 17, 1920.

5 "General Knowledge about Health, III," *Indian Opinion*, January 18, 1913.

6 Rathore, *Indian Political Theory*, 3; Gandhi, *A Guide to Health*; Gandhi, *Key to Health*; and "Note to Amrita Lal Chatterjee," April 15, 1941.

7 Flammang, *The Taste for Civilization*, 16; McClintock, *Imperial Leather*; and Stoler, *Carnal Knowledge and Imperial Power*.

8 Tidrick, *Gandhi*, 107; and Nayar, *Mahatma Gandhi*, 242–44.

9 Nandy, *The Intimate Enemy*, 48; Gandhi, "Loving Well," 93; Sinha, *Colonial Masculinity*; and Brumberg, *Fasting Girls*.

10 Brewer, "Savoring Time," 150; and "Letter to Sarladevi Chowdhrani," May 1, 1920.

11 "Letter to Sarladevi Chowdhrani," May 1, 1920; and Lal, "The Sexuality of a Celibate Life," 7.

12 "Letter to Sarladevi Chowdhrani," May 1, 1920.

13 "Letter to Sarladevi Chowdhrani," May 2, 1920; and Desmond, *Desire, Dialectic, and Otherness*, 83–84, 90.

14 "Letter to Sarladevi Chowdhrani," May 3, 1920.

Epigraph: "Raw v. Cooked Food," *Navajivan*, June 16, 1929.

1 It should be noted that many of Gandhi's colleagues did adjust their diet in the presence of the mahatma. For example, Vallabhbhai Patel told Mahadev Desai, "What is the use of taking tea after having become Bapu's companion in jail? I decided to eat exactly what he did. I gave up rice and take bread, milk and boiled vegetable like Bapu." See Desai, *Diary of Mahadev Desai*, 6. Also see Brown, *Gandhi's Rise to Power*, 42; and Guha, *Gandhi before India*, 545.

2 "Raw v. Cooked Food," *Navajivan*, June 16, 1929.

3 Saad, *The Global Hunger Crisis*.

4 Hassanein, "Practicing Food Democracy," 79; Douglas, "Deciphering a Meal," 80; Vodeb, *Food Democracy*; Kimura and Suryanata, *Food and Power in Hawai'i*; and Obach, *Organic Struggle*.

5 "Speech on 'Ashram Vows' at YMCA, Madras," February 16, 1916; and "General Knowledge about Health, IX," *Indian Opinion*, March 1, 1913.

6 Patel, *Stuffed and Starved*; Sainath, *Everybody Loves a Good Drought*; and Gray, *Labor and the Locavore*.

7 "Hindu-Mohammedan Unity," *Young India*, February 25, 1920; "Tea-Stalls," *Navajivan*, October 31, 1920; "Letter to G. K. Gokhale," June 7, 1913; "Food Faddists," *Young India*, June 13, 1929; "Speech at Muir College Economic Society, Allahabad," December 22, 1916; "Letter to V. S. Srinivasa Sastri," November 5, 1918; "Speech on Resolution on Office-Bearers, Belgaum Congress," December 27, 1924; "Letter to R. B. Gregg," April 26, 1927; and "Speech on Prohibition, Madras," September 6, 1927.

8 "Benevolent Parsis," *Navajivan*, September 15, 1921.

9 Friedman, "The Norwegian Military Is Fighting Climate Change"; and Bittman, *VB6*.

10 "Notes," *Young India*, February 2, 1922; Singer, *Animal Liberation*; Masson, *The Face on Your Plate*; and Foer, *Eating Animals*.

11 Institute of Governmental Studies, Proposition 2.

12 Maurer, *Vegetarianism*, 5 and 21.

13 Bégin, *Taste of the Nation*, 137; Johnston and Baumann, *Foodies*, 106–7. On the rich diversity of "Indian" food, see Achaya, *Indian Food*; Sen, *Food Culture in India*; Ray, "New Directions of Research on Indian Food"; Ray and Srinivas, *Curried Cultures*; and Appadurai, "How to Make a National Cuisine."

14 Slocum, "Race in the Study of Food," 27; Longhurst and Johnston, "Dishing Up Difference," 210; and Ganguly, "Global State of War and Moral Vernaculars of Nonviolence," 3.

15 "Letter to Esther Faering," January 29, 1920.

16 "General Knowledge about Health, IX," *Indian Opinion*, March 1, 1913.

17 "General Knowledge about Health, IX," *Indian Opinion*, March 1, 1913; and "Letter to Jamnadas Gandhi," May 30, 1913.

18 Fischler, "A Nutritional Cacophony"; and Erikson, *Gandhi's Truth*, 154.

Bibliography

Achaya, K. T. *Indian Food: A Historical Companion.* New York: Oxford University Press, 1994.

Alkon, Alison Hope, and Julian Agyeman, eds. *Cultivating Food Justice: Race, Class, and Sustainability.* Cambridge, MA: MIT Press, 2011.

Allinson, Thomas Richard. *The Advantages of Wholemeal Bread.* London: F. Pitman, 1889.

———. *Dr. Allinson's Cookery Book: Comprising Many Valuable Vegetarian Recipes.* www.gutenberg.org/ebooks/13887.

Alport, Susan. *Queen of Fats: Why Omega-3s Were Removed from the Western Diet and What We Can Do to Replace Them.* Berkeley: University of California Press, 2008.

Alter, Joseph S. *Gandhi's Body: Sex, Diet, and the Politics of Nationalism.* Philadelphia: University of Pennsylvania Press, 2000.

Ambedkar, Bhimrao Ramji. *What Congress and Gandhi Have Done to the Untouchables.* Bombay: Thacker, 1946.

Amin, Shahid. "Gandhi as Mahatma: Gorakhpur District, Eastern UP, 1921–2." In *Selected Subaltern Studies,* edited by Ranajit Guha and Gayatri Chakravorty Spivak, 288–348. New York: Oxford University Press, 1988.

Amsden, Matt, and Janabai Amsden. *The Rawvolution Continues: The Living Foods Movement in 150 Natural and Delicious Recipes.* New York: Atria Books, 2013.

Andrews, Geoff. *The Slow Food Story: Politics and Pleasure.* Montreal: McGill-Queen's University Press, 2008.

Anonymous. "Bread Reform League." *Journal of the Society of Arts* (May 13, 1881): 553.

———. *An Essay on Tea, Sugar, White Bread and Butter, Country Alehouses, Strong Beer and Geneva, and Other Modern Luxuries.* Salisbury, 1777.

———. "The Leader of the W.W.C.T.U. Food Reform Movement." *American Kitchen Magazine: A Domestic Science Monthly* 5 (1896): xiv.

Appadurai, Arjun. "How to Make a National Cuisine: Cookbooks in Contemporary India." *Comparative Studies in Society and History* 30, no. 1 (1988): 2–34.

Apple, Rima. *Vitamania: Vitamins in American Culture*. New Brunswick, NJ: Rutgers University Press, 1996.

Arnold, Carrie. *Decoding Anorexia: How Breakthroughs in Science Offer Hope for Eating Disorders*. New York: Routledge, 2012.

Arnold, David. "The Colonial Prison: Power, Knowledge and Penology in Nineteenth-Century India." In *Subaltern Studies VIII: Essays in Honour of Ranajit Guha*, edited by David Arnold and David Hardiman, 148–84. New Delhi: Oxford University Press, 1994.

——. *Colonizing the Body: State Medicine and Epidemic Disease in Nineteenth Century India*. Berkeley: University of California Press, 1993.

——. "The 'Discovery' of Malnutrition and Diet in Colonial India." *Indian Economic and Social History Review* 31, no. 1 (1994): 1–26.

——. *Gandhi: Profiles in Power*. New York: Routledge, 2001.

Aykroyd, Wallace Ruddell. "Beriberi and Other Food-Deficiency Diseases in Newfoundland and Labrador." *Journal of Hygiene* 30 (1930): 357–86.

——. *The Conquest of Famine*. New York: Reader's Digest Press, 1975.

——. "Nutrition and Public Health." *League of Nations Health Organization Quarterly Bulletin* 4 (1935): 323–474.

Banerjee, Sukanya. *Becoming Imperial Citizens: Indians in the Late-Victorian Empire*. Durham: Duke University Press, 2010.

Bardacke, Frank. *Trampling Out the Vintage: Cesar Chavez and the Two Souls of the United Farm Workers*. New York: Verso, 2011.

Bartlett, Rosamund. *Tolstoy: A Russian Life*. New York: Houghton Mifflin Harcourt, 2011.

Beauvoir, Simone de. *The Second Sex*. Translated by H. M. Parshley. New York: Vintage Books Edition, 1989.

Bégin, Camille. *Taste of the Nation: The New Deal Search for America's Food*. Urbana-Champaign, University of Illinois Press, 2016.

Belasco, Warren, and Philip Scranton, eds. *Food Nations: Selling Taste in Consumer Societies*. London: Routledge, 2002.

Berry, Wendell. *What Are People For? Essays*. Berkeley: Counterpoint, 2010.

Berson, Joshua. "The Quinoa Conundrum." *New Left Review* 85 (January–February 2014).

Bhana, Surendra, and Goolam Vahed, *The Making of a Political Reformer: Gandhi in South Africa, 1893–1914*. New Delhi: Manohar, 2005.

Bilgrami, Akeel. "Gandhi's Integrity: The Philosophy Behind the Politics." *Postcolonial Studies* 5, no. 1 (2002): 79–93.

Bittman, Mark. *VB6: Eat Vegan before 6:00 to Lose Weight and Restore Your Health . . . For Good*. New York: Clarkson Potter, 2013.

Black, Shameem. "Recipes for Cosmopolitanism: Cooking across Borders in the South Asian Diaspora." *Frontiers: A Journal of Women Studies* 31, no. 1 (2010): 1–30.

Bondurant, Joan. *Conquest of Violence: The Gandhian Philosophy of Conflict.* Princeton: Princeton University Press, 1998.

Brewer, Talbot. "Savoring Time: Desire, Pleasure and Wholehearted Activity." *Ethical Theory and Moral Practice* 6, no. 2 (2003): 143–60.

Brown, Judith M. *Gandhi's Rise to Power: Indian Politics 1915–1922.* Cambridge: Cambridge University Press, 1974.

Brown, Lester R. *Full Planet, Empty Plates: The New Geopolitics of Food Scarcity.* New York: Norton, 2012.

Brumberg, Joan Jacobs. *Fasting Girls: The History of Anorexia Nervosa.* Cambridge, MA: Harvard University Press, 1988.

Bryant, Edwin. "Strategies of Vedic Subversion: The Emergence of Vegetarianism in Post-Vedic India." In *A Communion of Subjects: Animals in Religion, Science, and Ethics,* edited by Paul Waldau and Kimberley C. Patton, 194–203. New York: Columbia University Press, 2009.

Burton, David. *The Raj at Table.* London: Faber and Faber, 1993.

Butterly, John R., and Jack Shepherd. *Hunger: The Biology and Politics of Starvation.* Hanover, NH: Dartmouth College Press, 2010.

Bynum, Caroline Walker. *Holy Feast and Holy Fast: The Religious Significance of Food to Medieval Women.* Berkeley: University of California Press, 1988.

Cannon, Geoffrey, and Claus Leitzmann. "The New Nutrition Science Project." *Public Health Nutrition* 8, no. 6a (2005): 673–94.

Cappeliez, Sarah, and Josée Johnston. "From Meat and Potatoes to 'Real-Deal' Rotis: Exploring Everyday Culinary Cosmopolitanism." *Poetics* 41, no. 5 (2013): 433–55.

Carpenter, Kenneth. *Beriberi, White Rice, and Vitamin B.* Berkeley: University of California Press, 2000.

———. "The Work of Wallace Aykroyd: International Nutritionist and Author." *Journal of Nutrition* 137, no. 4 (2007): 873–78.

Chapple, Christopher Key. *Jainism and Ecology: Nonviolence in the Web of Life.* Center for the Study of World Religions, 2002.

Chatterjee, Manini. "1930: Turning Point in the Participation of Women in the Freedom Struggle." *Social Scientist* 29, no. 7/8 (2001): 39–47.

Chatterjee, Piya. *A Time for Tea: Women, Labor, and Post/Colonial Politics on an Indian Plantation.* Durham: Duke University Press, 2001.

Collingham, E. M. *Imperial Bodies: The Physical Experience of the Raj, c. 1800–1947.* Cambridge: Polity, 2001.

Collingham, Lizzie. *Curry: A Tale of Cooks and Conquerors.* Oxford: Oxford University Press, 2007.

Conford, Philip. *The Origins of the Organic Movement.* Edinburgh: Floris Books, 2001.

Connelly, Matthew. *Fatal Misconception: The Struggle to Control World Population.* Cambridge, MA: Belknap Press, 2010.

Cordain, Loren. *The Paleo Diet: Lose Weight and Get Healthy by Eating the Foods You Were Designed to Eat*. Hoboken: John Wiley & Sons, 2002.

Cordain, Loren, and T. Colin Campbell. "The Protein Debate." *Performance Menu: Journal of Nutrition and Athletic Excellence*.

Cordain, Loren, S. Boyd Eaton, et al. "Origins and Evolution of the Western Diet: Health Implications for the Twenty-First Century." *American Journal of Clinical Nutrition* 81, no. 2 (2005): 341–54.

Corman, Lauren. "The Ventriloquist's Burden: Animal Advocacy and the Problem of Speaking for Others." In *Animal Subjects 2.0*, edited by Jodey Castricano and Lauren Corman, 473–512. Waterloo: Wilfrid Laurier University Press, 2016.

Cort, John E. *Jains in the World: Religious Values and Ideology in India*. Oxford: Oxford University Press, 2001.

———. "Singing the Glory of Asceticism: Devotion of Asceticism in Jainism." *Journal of the American Academy of Religion* 70, no. 4 (2002): 719–42.

Crosby, Alfred W. *The Columbian Exchange: Biological and Cultural Consequences of 1492*. Westport, CT: Greenwood Publishing, 1972.

Dalton, Dennis. *Mahatma Gandhi: Nonviolent Power in Action*. New York: Columbia University Press, 2000.

Das Gupta, A. K. *Gandhi's Economic Thought*. London: Routledge, 1996.

Davis, Mike. *Late Victorian Holocausts: El Niño Famines and the Making of the Third World*. New York: Verso, 2002.

Davis, R. Hunt, Jr.. "John L. Dube: A South African Exponent of Booker T. Washington." *Journal of African Studies* 2, no. 4 (1975–1976): 497–528.

de la Peña, Carolyn. *Empty Pleasures: The Story of Artificial Sweeteners from Saccharin to Splenda*. Chapel Hill: University of North Carolina Press, 2012.

Desai, Ashwin, and Goolam Vahed, *The South African Gandhi: Stretcher-Bearer of Empire*. New Delhi: Navayana, 2015.

Desai, Mahadev. *Diary of Mahadev Desai*. Vol. 1. Ahmedabad: Navajivan, 1953.

Desmond, William. *Desire, Dialectic, and Otherness: An Essay on Origins*, Second Edition. Eugene, OR: Cascade, 2013.

Digby, A., W. Ernst, and P. B. Muhkarji, eds. *Crossing Colonial Historiographies: Histories of Colonial and Indigenous Medicines in Transnational Perspective*. Cambridge: Cambridge University Press, 2010.

Djousse, Luc, and J. Michael Gaziano. "Egg Consumption in Relation to Cardiovascular Disease and Mortality: The Physician's Health Study." *American Journal of Clinical Nutrition* 87 (2008): 964–69.

Doctor, Vikram. "Purslane: India's Gift to the World." *Economic Times*, May 27, 2011.

Dombrowski, Daniel A. *The Philosophy of Vegetarianism*. Amherst: University of Massachusetts Press, 1984.

Dosanjh, Ujjal. "Cow Vigilantism Threatens the Body and Soul of India." *Indian Express*, April 16, 2017.

Douglas, Mary. "Deciphering a Meal." *Daedalus* 101, no. 1 (1972): 61–81.

———. *"Purity and Danger: An Analysis of Concepts of Pollution and Taboo*. New York: Routledge, 1966.

Drayton, Richard. *Nature's Government: Science, Imperial Britain, and the "Improvement" of the World*. New Haven: Yale University Press, 2000.

Dundas, Paul. *The Jains*, Second Edition. New York: Routledge, 2002.

Dupuis, E. Melanie. *Nature's Perfect Food: How Milk Became America's Drink*. New York: NYU Press, 2002.

Dutt, Rajani Palme. "Rajani Palme Dutt: An Indian Communist's View from Britain." In *Sources of Indian Tradition: Modern India, Pakistan, and Bangladesh*, edited by Rachel Fell McDermott, Leonard A. Gordon, Ainslie T. Embree, Frances W. Pritchett, and Dennis Dalton, 402–7. New York: Columbia University Press, 2014.

Dutt, Romesh Chunder. *The Economic History of India in the Victorian Age*. London: Routledge, 1950.

Eck, Diana L. *Darśan: Seeing the Divine Image in India*. New York: Columbia University Press, 1998.

Elwood, Anne Katherine Curteis. *Narrative of a Journey Overland from England, by the Continent of Europe, Egypt and the Red Sea to India Including a Residence There, and Voyage Home, in the Years 1825, 26, 27, and 28, vol. 1*. London: H. Colburn & Richard Bentley, 1830.

Erikson, Erik H. *Gandhi's Truth: On the Origins of Militant Nonviolence*. New York: W. W. Norton & Company, 1970.

Fischler, Claude. "A Nutritional Cacophony or the Crisis of Food Selection in Affluent Societies." In *For a Better Nutrition in the 21st Century*, edited by P. Leathwood, M. Horisberger, and W. James, 57–65. New York: Vevey/Raven Press, 1993.

Flammang, Janet A. *The Taste for Civilization: Food, Politics, and Civil Society*. Urbana-Champaign: The University of Illinois Press, 2009.

Foer, Jonathan Safran. *Eating Animals*. Boston: Back Bay Books, 2010.

Forward, Charles Walter. *Fifty Years of Food Reform: A History of the Vegetarian Movement in England*. London: Ideal Publishing Union, 1898.

Freidberg, Susanne. *Fresh: A Perishable History*. Cambridge, MA: Belknap Press, 2009.

Friedman, Uri. "The Norwegian Military Is Fighting Climate Change with 'Meatless Mondays.'" *Atlantic*, November 21, 2013.

Gandhi, Leela. "Ahimsa and Other Animals: The Genealogy of an Immature Politics." *Borderlands* 4, no. 3 (2005). www.borderlands.net.au/vol4no3_2005/gandhi_ahimsa.htm.

———. "Loving Well: Homosexuality and Utopian Thought in Post/Colonial India." In *Queering India: Same-Sex Love and Eroticism in Indian Culture and Society*, edited by Ruth Vanita, 87–99. New York: Routledge, 2002.

Gandhi, Mohandas K. *An Autobiography: The Story of My Experiments with Truth.* Ahmedabad: Navajivan, 1996.

———. *The Collected Works of Mahatma Gandhi.* New Delhi: Publications Division, Ministry of Information and Broadcasting, Government of India, 1958–1994.

———. *The Collected Works of Mahatma Gandhi.* Electronic book. New Delhi: Publications Division, Government of India, 1999. This edition is cited in notes, abbreviated *CWMG.*

———. *A Guide to Health.* Madras: S. Ganesan, 1921.

———. *Hind Swaraj.* Ahmedabad: Navajivan, 1938. Available at www.mkgandhi .org/ebks/hind_swaraj.pdf.

———. *Key to Health.* Edited by Jitendra T. Desai. Ahmedabad: Navajivan, 1948.

———. *Satyagraha in South Africa.* Ahmedabad: Navajivan, 1968.

Gandhi, Rajmohan. *The Good Boatman: A Portrait of Gandhi.* New Delhi: Penguin, 1995.

———. *Mohandas: A True Story of a Man, His People and an Empire.* New York: Penguin, 2007.

Ganguly, Debjani. "Global State of War and Moral Vernaculars of Nonviolence: Rethinking Gandhi in a New World Order." In *Rethinking Gandhi and Nonviolent Relationality Global Perspectives*, edited by Debjani Ganguly and John Docker, 1–14. London: Routledge, 2007.

Garcia, Matthew. *From the Jaws of Victory: The Triumph and Tragedy of Cesar Chavez and the Farm Worker Movement.* Berkeley: University of California Press, 2012.

Graham, Sylvester. *Treatise on Bread and Bread-Making.* Boston: Light & Stearns, 1837.

Gottlieb, Robert, and Anupama Joshi, eds. *Food Justice.* Cambridge, MA: MIT Press, 2013.

Grant, Kevin. "British Suffragettes and the Russian Method of Hunger Strike." *Comparative Studies in Society and History* 53, no. 1 (2011): 113–43.

Gray, Margaret. *Labor and the Locavore: The Making of a Comprehensive Food Ethic.* Berkeley: University of California Press, 2013.

Green, Martin B. *Gandhi: Voice of a New Age Revolution.* Mount Jackson, VA: Axios Press, 1993.

Green, Nile. "Kebabs and Port Wine: The Culinary Cosmopolitanism of Anglo-Persian Dining, 1800–1835." In *Cosmopolitanisms in Muslim Contexts: Perspectives from the Past*, edited by Derryl N. MacLean and Sikeena Karmali Ahmed, 105–26. Edinburgh: Edinburgh University Press, 2013.

Gregory, James. *Of Victorians and Vegetarians: The Vegetarian Movement in Nineteenth-Century Britain*. London: I. B. Tauris, 2007.

Guha, Ramachandra. *Gandhi before India*. New York: Knopf, 2014.

Guha, Ranajit. *Dominance without Hegemony: History and Power in Colonial India*. Cambridge, MA: Harvard University Press, 1998.

Guthman, Julie. "Commentary on Teaching Food: Why I Am Fed Up with Michael Pollan et al." *Agriculture and Human Values* 24 (2007): 261–64.

———. *Weighing In: Obesity, Food Justice, and the Limits of Capitalism*. Berkeley: University of California Press, 2011.

Hajari, Nisid. *Midnight's Furies: The Deadly Legacy of India's Partition*. New York: Houghton Mifflin Harcourt, 2015.

Haller, John S. *The History of Homeopathy: The Academic Years, 1820–1935*. New Brunswick, NJ: Rutgers University Press, 2005.

Hamilton, Lisa M. "The Quinoa Quarrel: Who Owns the World's Greatest Superfood?" *Harper's* (May 2014): 35–42.

Hardiman, David. *Gandhi in His Time and Ours: The Global Legacy of His Ideas*. New York: Columbia University Press, 2004.

Harrison, Mark. *Climates and Constitutions: Health, Race, Environment and British Imperialism in India, 1600–1850*. Delhi: Oxford University Press, 1999.

Hassanein, Neva. "Practicing Food Democracy: A Pragmatic Politics of Transformation." *Journal of Rural Studies* 19, no. 1 (2003): 77–86.

Hauter, Wenonah. *Foodopoly: The Battle over the Future of Food and Farming in America*. New York: New Press, 2012.

Hay, Stephen. "The Making of a Late-Victorian Hindu: M. K. Gandhi in London, 1888–1891." *Victorian Studies* 33, no. 1 (1989): 75–98.

Hayes, J. D., M. O. Kelleher, and I. M. Eggleston. "The Cancer Chemopreventive Actions of Phytochemicals Derived from Glucosinolates." *European Journal of Nutrition* 47, no. 2 (2008): 73–88.

Heldke, Lisa. *Exotic Appetites: Ruminations of a Food Adventurer*. New York: Routledge, 2003.

Hendrick, George. *Henry Salt: Humanitarian Reformer and Man of Letters*. Urbana: University of Illinois Press, 1977.

Hendrick, George, and Willene Hendrick, eds. *The Savour of Salt: A Henry Salt Anthology*. Fontwell, Sussex: Centaur Press, 1999.

Hendricks, Steve. "Starving Your Way to Vigor: The Benefits of an Empty Stomach." *Harper's* (March 2012): 27–38.

Herman, Arthur. *Gandhi and Churchill: The Epic Rivalry That Destroyed an Empire and Forged Our Age*. New York: Bantam, 2009.

Herring, Ronald J. *Land to the Tiller: The Political Economy of Agrarian Reform in South Asia*. New Haven: Yale University Press, 1983.

Hesterman, Oran B. *Fair Food: Growing a Healthy, Sustainable Food System for All.* New York: PublicAffairs, 2011.

Hills, Arnold. "The Vegetarian Federal Union: Its Possibilities and Its Policy." *Vegetarian*, December 21, 1889.

Hobart, Hi'ilei Julia. "A 'Queer-Looking Compound': Race, Abjection, and the Politics of Hawaiian Poi." *Global Food History* 3, no. 2 (2017): 133–49.

Hofmeyr, Isabel. *Gandhi's Printing Press: Experiments in Slow Reading.* Cambridge, MA: Harvard University Press, 2013.

Holt-Giménez, Eric, ed. *Food Movements Unite! Strategies to Transform Our Food Systems.* Oakland: Food First Books, 2011.

Hunt, James D. "Gandhi and the Black People of South Africa." Website of the Bombay Sarvodaya Mandal and the Gandhi Research Foundation. www.mkgandhi.org/articles/jamesdhunt.htm.

———. *Gandhi in London.* New Delhi: Promilla, 1978.

Iacobbo, Karen, and Michael Iacobbo. *Vegetarian America: A History.* Westport, CT: Praeger, 2004.

Institute of Governmental Studies. Proposition 2. IGS, University of California, Berkeley. https://igs.berkeley.edu/library/elections/proposition-2.

Jaffrelot, Christophe. *Dr. Ambedkar and Untouchability: Fighting the Indian Caste System.* New York: Columbia University Press, 2005.

Jhala, Angma D. "Cosmopolitan Kitchens: Cooking for Princely Zenanas in Late Colonial India." In *Curried Cultures: Globalization, Food, and South Asia*, edited by Krishnendu Ray and Tulasi Srinivas, 49–72. Berkeley: University of California Press, 2012.

Johnson, Samuel, and James Boswell. *A Journey to the Western Islands of Scotland and the Journal of a Tour to the Hebrides.* London: Penguin, 1984.

Johnston, Josée, and Shyon Baumann. *Foodies: Democracy and Distinction in the Gourmet Foodscape.* New York: Routledge, 2009.

Jordens, J. T. F. *Gandhi's Religion: A Homespun Shawl.* New York: Palgrave Macmillan, 1998.

Kaelber, Walter O. "'Tapas,' Birth, and Spiritual Rebirth in the Veda." *History of Religions* 15, no. 4 (1976): 343–86.

Kale, Madhavi. *Fragments of Empire: Capital, Slavery, and Indian Indentured Labor Migration in the British Caribbean.* Philadelphia: University of Pennsylvania Press, 1998.

Katz, Esther, ed. *The Selected Papers of Margaret Sanger.* Vol. 4, *'Round the World for Birth Control (1920–1966).* Urbana: University of Illinois Press, 2016.

Kaufman, Frederick. *Bet the Farm: How Food Stopped Being Food.* Hoboken: Wiley, 2012.

Kaufman, Martin. *Homeopathy in America: The Rise and Fall of a Medical Heresy.* Baltimore: Johns Hopkins Press, 1971.

Kenney, Matthew. *Cooked Raw: How One Celebrity Chef Risked Everything to Change the Way We Eat*. Familius, 2015.

Khan, Yasmin. *The Great Partition: The Making of India and Pakistan*. New Haven: Yale University Press, 2007.

Kimura, Aya Hirata, and Krisnawati Suryanata, eds. *Food and Power in Hawai'i: Visions of Food Democracy*. Manoa: University of Hawai'i Press, 2016.

King, Martin Luther. *The Papers of Martin Luther King, Jr.* Vol. 5, *Threshold of a New Decade, January 1959–December 1960*. Edited by Clayborne Carson, Tenisha Armstrong, Susan Carson, Adrienne Clay, and Kieran Taylor. Berkeley: University of California Press, 2005.

King, Mary Elizabeth. *Gandhian Nonviolent Struggle and Untouchability in South India: The 1924–25 Vykom Satyagraha and the Mechanisms of Change*. Delhi: Oxford University Press, 2015.

Kingsford, Anna. *The Perfect Way in Diet: A Treatise Advocating a Return to the Natural and Ancient Food of Our Race*. London: Kegan Paul, Trench, Trubner and Co., 1895.

Kipling, Rudyard. "William the Conqueror—Part II." From *The Day's Work*. https://ebooks.adelaide.edu.au/k/kipling/rudyard/days/chapter7.html.

Kishwar, Madhu. "Gandhi and Women." *Economic and Political Weekly* 20 (October 5, 1985 and October 12, 1985): 1691–1702 and 1753–58.

Kivelä, A. M., et al. "Sulforaphane Inhibits Endothelial Lipase Expression through NF-κB in Endothelial Cells." *Atherosclerosis* 213, no. 1 (2010): 122–28.

Kosek, Joseph Kip. "Richard Gregg, Mohandas Gandhi, and the Strategy of Nonviolence." *Journal of American History* 91, no. 4 (2005): 1318–48.

Krondi, Michael. "The Sweetshops of Kolkata." *Gastronomica: The Journal of Food and Culture* 10, no. 3 (2010): 58–65.

Kumar, Aishwary. *Radical Equality: Ambedkar, Gandhi, and the Risk of Democracy*. Stanford: Stanford University Press, 2015.

Kurlansky, Mark. *Salt: A World History*. New York: Penguin, 2003.

Laidlaw, James. "A Life Worth Leaving: Fasting to Death as Telos of a Jain Religious Life." *Economy and Society* 34, no. 2 (2005): 178–99.

———. *Riches and Renunciation: Religion, Economy, and Society among the Jains*. Oxford: Clarendon Press, 1996.

Lal, Vinay. "Nakedness, Nonviolence, and Brahmacharya: Gandhi's Experiments in Celibate Sexuality." *Journal of the History of Sexuality* 9, nos. 1–2 (2000): 105–36.

———. "The Sexuality of a Celibate Life." *Asian Age*, May 1, 2011.

Lal, Vinay, and Ellen DuBois, eds. *A Passionate Life: Writings by and on Kamladevi Chattopadhyay*. New Delhi: Zubaan Books, 2017.

Langford, Jean M. *Fluent Bodies: Ayurvedic Remedies for Postcolonial Imbalance*. Durham: Duke University Press, 2002.

Larson, N. I., M. T. Story, and M. C. Nelson. "Neighborhood Environments: Disparities in Access to Healthy Foods in the U.S." *American Journal of Preventive Medicine* 36, no. 1 (2009): 74–81.

Laszlo, Pierre. *Salt: Grain of Life*. New York: Columbia University Press, 2001.

Laudan, Rachel. *Cuisine and Empire: Cooking in World History*. Berkeley: University of California Press, 2013.

Lavrin, Janko. "Tolstoy and Gandhi." *Russian Review* 19, no. 2 (1960): 132–39.

Lelyveld, Joseph. *Great Soul: Mahatma Gandhi and His Struggle With India*. New York: Knopf, 2011.

Leong-Salobir, Cecilia. *Food Culture in Colonial Asia: A Taste of Empire*. New York: Routledge, 2011.

Levenstein, Harvey A. *Revolution at the Table: The Transformation of the American Diet*. New York: Oxford University Press, 1988.

Lévi-Strauss, Claude. *The Raw and the Cooked: Mythologiques*. Vol. 1. Chicago: University of Chicago Press, 1983.

Lichtenstein, Alice, and Robert Russell. "Essential Nutrients: Food or Supplements? Where Should the Emphasis Be?" *Journal of the American Medical Association* 294, no. 3 (2005): 351–58.

Lobel, Cindy. "Sylvester Graham and Antebellum Diet Reform." *History Now*. www.gilderlehrman.org/history-now/sylvester-graham-and-antebellum-diet -reform.

Lockeretz, William, ed. *Organic Farming: An International History*. Wallingford: CABI, 2007.

Long, Jeffery D. *Jainism: An Introduction*. London: I. B. Tauris, 2009.

Longhurst, Robyn, and Lynda Johnston. "Dishing Up Difference: Assemblages of Food, Home and Migrant Women in Hamilton, Aotearoa New Zealand." In *Geographies of Race and Food: Fields, Bodies, Markets*, edited by Rachel Slocum and Arun Saldanha, 199–216. New York: Routledge, 2016.

Mahias, Marie-Claude. "Milk and Its Transmutations in Indian Society." *Food and Foodways* 2, no. 1 (1987): 265–88.

Maine, Henry Sumner. *Village-Communities in the East and West*. London: John Murray, 1871.

Mannur, Anita. *Culinary Fictions: Food in South Asian Diasporic Culture*. Philadelphia: Temple University Press, 2009.

Mantena, Karuna. *Alibis of Empire: Henry Maine and the Ends of Liberal Imperialism*. Princeton: Princeton University Press, 2010.

Marable, William Manning. *African Nationalist: The Life of John Langalibalele Dube*. Michigan: UMI Dissertation Services, 1976.

Margaret Sanger Papers Project. "Gandhi and Sanger Debate Love, Lust and Birth Control." Newsletter #23 (winter 1999–2000). www.nyu.edu/projects /sanger/articles/gandhi_debate.php.

Markovits, Claude. *The Ungandhian-Gandhi: The Life and Afterlife of the Mahatma*. London: Anthem Press, 2003.

Maroney, Stephanie R. "'To Make a Curry the India Way': Tracking the Meaning of Curry Across Eighteenth-Century Communities." *Food and Foodways* 19, nos. 1–2 (2011): 122–34.

Masson, Jeffrey Moussaieff. *The Face on Your Plate*. New York: W. W. Norton, 2009.

Maurer, Donna. *Vegetarianism: Movement or Moment?* Philadelphia: Temple University Press, 2002.

Mazumdar, Sucheta. "The Impact of New World Food Crops on the Diet and Economy of China and India, 1600–1900." In *Food and Global History*, edited by Raymond Grew, 58–78. Boulder, CO: Westview Press, 1999.

McCarrison, Robert. "A Good Diet and a Bad One: An Experimental Contrast." *British Medical Journal* 2 (October 23, 1926): 730–32.

———. "Nutrition in Health and Disease." *British Medical Journal* 2 (1936): 611.

———. "Problems of Nutrition in India." In *The Work of Sir Robert McCarrison*, edited by H. M. Sinclair, 267–68. London: Faber & Faber, 1953.

———. "The Relation of Manure to the Nutritive and Vitamin Value of Certain Grain." *British Medical Journal* 1 (March 29, 1924): 567–69.

McCay, David. *The Protein Element in Nutrition*. London: E. Arnold, 1912.

McClintock, Anne. *Imperial Leather: Race, Gender, and Sexuality in the Colonial Contest*. New York: Routledge, 1995.

McKeogh, Colm. *Tolstoy's Pacifism*. Amherst: Cambria Press, 2009.

Mehta, Ved. *Mahatma Gandhi and His Apostles*. New Haven: Yale University Press, 1993.

Mente, Andrew, et al. "Association of Urinary Sodium and Potassium Excretion with Blood Pressure." *New England Journal of Medicine* 371 (2014): 601–11.

Merton, Thomas. "Gandhi and the One-Eyed Giant." In *Gandhi on Nonviolence*, 3–34. New York: New Directions, 1965.

Metcalf, Thomas R. *Imperial Connections: India in the Indian Ocean Arena, 1860–1920*. Berkeley: University of California Press, 2007.

Meyer-Renschausen, Elisabeth. "The Porridge Debate: Grain, Nutrition, and Forgotten Food Preparation Techniques." *Food and Foodways* 5, no. 1 (1991): 95–120.

Miller, Webb. *I Found No Peace*. New York: Simon and Schuster, 1936.

Mintz, Sidney. *Sweetness and Power: The Place of Sugar in Modern History*. New York: Penguin, 1985.

———. *Tasting Food, Tasting Freedom: Excursions into Eating, Culture, and the Past*. Boston: Beacon Press, 1996.

Moss, Michael. *Salt, Sugar, Fat: How the Food Giants Hooked Us*. New York: Random House, 2013.

Moxham, Roy. "Salt Starvation in British India: Consequences of High Salt Taxation in Bengal Presidency, 1765 to 1878." *Economic and Political Weekly* 36, no. 25 (2001): 2270–74.

Mozaffarian, Dariush, et al. "Global Sodium Consumption and Death from Cardiovascular Causes." *New England Journal of Medicine* 371 (2014): 624–34.

Mukerjee, Madhusree. *Churchill's Secret War: The British Empire and the Ravaging of India During World War II.* New York: Basic Books, 2011.

Murillo, G., and R. G. Mehta. "Cruciferous Vegetables and Cancer Prevention." *Nutrition and Cancer* 41, nos. 1–2 (2001): 17–28.

Murthy, B. Srinivasa. *Mahatma Gandhi and Leo Tolstoy Letters.* Long Beach, CA: Long Beach Publications, 1987.

Nagaraj, D. R. *The Flaming Feet and Other Essays: The Dalit Movement in India.* Edited by Prithvi Datta Chandra Shobhi. Chicago: University of Chicago Press, 2010.

Nanda, B. R. *In Search of Gandhi.* Oxford: Oxford University Press, 2002.

———. *Mahatma Gandhi: A Biography.* Delhi: Oxford India, 1996.

Nanda, Reena. *Kamaladevi Chattopadhyay: A Biography.* New Delhi: Oxford, 2002.

Nandy, Ashish. "Final Encounter: The Politics of the Assassination of Gandhi." In *At the Edge of Psychology: Essays in Politics and Culture*, by Ashish Nandy, 70–99. Delhi: Oxford University Press, 1980.

———. *The Intimate Enemy: Loss and Recovery of Self under Colonialism.* Delhi: Oxford University Press, 1983.

Narasimhan, Sakuntala. *Kamaladevi Chattopadhyay: The Romantic Rebel.* New Delhi: Sterling, 1999.

Narayan, Uma. *Dislocating Cultures: Identities, Traditions, and Third World Feminism.* New York: Routledge, 1997.

Nauriya, Anil. *The African Element in Gandhi.* New Delhi: National Gandhi Museum, 2006.

Nayar, Pramod K. *Packaging Life: Cultures of the Everyday.* Thousand Oaks, CA: Sage, 2009.

Nayar, Sushila. *Mahatma Gandhi.* Ahmedabad: 1994.

Naylor, Rosamond L., ed. *The Evolving Sphere of Food Security.* Oxford: Oxford University Press, 2014.

Nestle, Marion. *Food Politics: How the Food Industry Influences Nutrition and Health.* Berkeley: University of California Press, 2003.

———. "Paleolithic Diets: A Sceptical View." *British Nutrition Foundation* 25 (2000): 43–47.

Norton, Marcy. "Tasting Empire: Chocolate and the European Internalization of Mesoamerican Aesthetics." *American Historical Review* 111 (2006): 660–91.

Obach, Brian K. *Organic Struggle: The Movement for Sustainable Agriculture in the United States.* Cambridge, MA: MIT Press, 2015.

O'Donnell, Martin, et al. "Urinary Sodium and Potassium Excretion, Mortality, and Cardiovascular Events." *New England Journal of Medicine* 371 (2014): 612–23.

Oldfield, Josiah. "My Friend Gandhi." In *Reminiscences of Gandhiji*, edited by Chandrashanker Shukla, 187–88. Bombay: Vora and Co., 1951.

Patel, Raj. *Stuffed and Starved: The Hidden Battle for the World Food System.* Brooklyn: Melville House, 2012.

Pawel, Miriam. *The Union of Their Dreams: Power, Hope, and Struggle in Cesar Chavez's Farm Worker Movement.* New York: Bloomsbury, 2010.

Pearson, Anne Mackenzie. *Because It Gives Me Peace of Mind: Ritual Fasts in the Religious Lives of Hindu Women.* Albany: State University of New York Press, 1996.

Penniman, Leah. "Radical Farmers Use Fresh Food to Fight Racial Injustice and the New Jim Crow." *Yes!* September 5, 2015.

Petrini, Carlo. *Slow Food: The Case for Taste*, translated by William McCuaig. New York: Columbia University Press, 2004.

Pföstl, Eva. *Between Ethics and Politics: New Essays on Gandhi.* New Delhi: Routledge, 2014.

Plimmer, Robert Henry Aders, and Violet Geraldine Sheffield Plimmer. *Food, Health, Vitamins; Being a New Edition of Food and Health.* London: Longmans, Green and Co., 1926.

Pokorski, Robin. "Sanger and Gandhi: A Complex Relationship." Margaret Sanger Papers Project, October 2, 2013. https://sangerpapers.wordpress.com/2013/10/02/sanger-and-gandhi-a-complex-relationship.

Polak, Millie Graham. *Mr. Gandhi: The Man.* London: George Allen and Unwin, 1931.

Pollan, Michael. *Cooked: A Natural History of Transformation.* New York: Penguin, 2013.

———. *In Defense of Food: The Myth of Nutrition and the Pleasures of Eating.* New York: Penguin, 2008.

Prasad, Rajendra. *Satyagraha in Champaran.* Ahmedabad: Navajivan, 1949.

Preece, Rod. *Sins of the Flesh: A History of Ethical Vegetarian Thought.* Vancouver: UBC Press, 2009.

Rathore, Aakash Singh. *Indian Political Theory: Laying the Groundwork for Svaraj.* New York: Routledge, 2017.

Ray, Bharati. *Early Feminists of Colonial India: Sarala Devi Chaudhurani and Rokeya Sakhawat Hossain.* New Delhi: Oxford University Press, 2002.

Ray, Krishnendu. *The Ethnic Restaurateur.* London: Bloomsbury, 2016.

———. *The Migrant's Table: Meals and Memories in Bengali-American Households.* Philadelphia: Temple University Press, 2004.

———. "New Directions of Research on Indian Food." In *Writing Food History: A Global Perspective*, edited by Kyri W. Claflin and Peter Scholliers, 165–80. London: Berg, 2012.

Ray, Krishnendu, and Tulasi Srinivas, eds. *Curried Cultures: Globalization, Food, and South Asia.* Berkeley: University of California Press, 2012.

Robidoux, Michael A., and Courtney W. Mason, eds. *A Land Not Forgotten: Indigenous Food Security and Land-Based Practices in Northern Ontario.* Winnipeg: University of Manitoba Press, 2017.

Rothermund, Dietmar. *An Economic History of India.* New York: Routledge, 1993.

Roy, Parama. *Alimentary Tracts: Appetites, Aversions, and the Postcolonial.* Durham: Duke University Press, 2010.

Saad, Majda Bne. *The Global Hunger Crisis: Tackling Food Insecurity in Developing Countries.* London: Pluto Press, 2013.

Safi, Michael. "Muslim Man Dies in India after Attack by Hindu 'Cow Protectors.'" *Guardian*, April 5, 2017.

Sainath, Palagummi. *Everybody Loves a Good Drought: Stories from India's Poorest Districts.* New York: Penguin Books, 1996.

Salatin, Joel. *Everything I Want to Do Is Illegal: War Stories from the Local Food Front.* Polyface, 2007.

Salt, Henry S. *Animals' Rights: Considered in Relation to Social Progress.* New York: Macmillan and Co., 1894.

———. *The Logic of Vegetarianism: Essays and Dialogues.* London: George Bell and Sons, 1906.

Sanger, Margaret. "Does Mr. Gandhi Know Women?" *Illustrated Weekly of India*, January 19, 1936.

Sapolsky, Robert. *Why Zebras Don't Get Ulcers.* New York: Holt, 2004.

Schubert, Lisa, et al. "Re-imagining the 'Social' in the Nutrition Sciences." *Public Health Nutrition* 15, no. 2 (2011): 352–59.

Scrinis, Gyorgy. *Nutritionism: The Science and Politics of Dietary Advice.* New York: Columbia University Press, 2013.

Sen, Amartya. *Poverty and Famines: An Essay on Entitlement and Deprivation.* Oxford: Clarendon Press, 1982.

Sen, Arijit. "Food, Place, and Memory: Bangladeshi Fish Stores on Devon Avenue, Chicago." *Food and Foodways* 24, nos. 1–2 (2016): 67–88.

Sen, Colleen Taylor. *Food Culture in India.* Westport, CT: Greenwood, 2004.

Shanti, George. *Operation Flood: An Appraisal of Current Indian Dairy Policy.* Delhi: Oxford University Press, 1985.

Shapiro, Laura. *Perfection Salad: Women and Cooking at the Turn of the Century.* New York: Farrar, Straus, and Giroux, 1986.

Sharma, Arvind. *Gandhi: A Spiritual Biography*. New Haven: Yale University Press, 2013.

Sharma, Jayeeta. "Food and Empire." In *Oxford Handbook of Food History*, edited by Jeffrey M. Pilcher, 241–57. New York: Oxford University Press, 2012.

Shelley, Percy Bysshe. *The Complete Poetical Works of Shelley*. Boston: Houghton Mifflin Company, 1901.

Shenker, Israel. "E. B. White: Notes and Comment by Author." *New York Times*, July 11, 1969.

Shetty, Sandhya. "The Quack Whom We Know: Illness and Nursing in Gandhi." In *Rethinking Gandhi and Nonviolent Relationality: Global Perspectives*, edited by Debjani Ganguly and John Docker, 38–65. London: Routledge, 2007.

Sholten, Bruce A. *India's White Revolution: Operation Flood, Food Aid and Development*. London: Tauris Academic Studies, 2010.

Shprintzen, Adam D. *The Vegetarian Crusade: The Rise of an American Reform Movement, 1817–1921*. Chapel Hill: University of North Carolina Press, 2013.

Sifferlin, Alexandra. "Salt Sugar Fat: Q&A with Author Michael Moss." *Time*, February 26, 2013. http://healthland.time.com/2013/02/26/salt-sugar-fat-qa -with-author-michael-moss.

Singer, Peter. *Animal Liberation: Towards an End to Man's Inhumanity to Animals*. New York: HarperCollins, 1975.

——. *The Most Good You Can Do: How Effective Altruism Is Changing Ideas about Living Ethically*. New Haven: Yale University Press, 2015.

Sinha, Mrinalini. *Colonial Masculinity: The 'Manly Englishman' and the 'Effeminate Bengali' in the Late Nineteenth Century*. Manchester: Manchester University Press, 1995.

Skaria, Ajay. *Unconditional Equality: Gandhi's Religion of Resistance*. Minneapolis: University of Minnesota Press, 2016.

Slate, Nico. *Colored Cosmopolitanism: The Shared Struggle for Freedom in the United States and India*. Cambridge, MA: Harvard University Press, 2012.

——. "From Mealie Pap to Peanut Milk: The African Diaspora, Culinary Cosmopolitanism, and Mahatma Gandhi's Evolving Views on Race and Diet." Under review at *Global Food History*.

Slocum, Rachel. "Race in the Study of Food." In *Geographies of Race and Food: Fields, Bodies, Markets*, edited by Rachel Slocum and Arun Saldanha, 25–60. New York: Routledge, 2016.

Smith-Howard, Kendra. *Pure and Modern Milk: An Environmental History Since 1900*. New York: Oxford University Press, 2013.

Soluri, John. *Banana Cultures: Agriculture, Consumption, and Environmental Change in Honduras and the United States*. Austin: University of Texas Press, 2006.

Spencer, Colin. *Vegetarianism: A History*. New York: Da Capo Press, 2004.

Stacey, Michelle. *Consumed: Why Americans Love, Hate and Fear Food*. New York: Simon and Schuster, 1994.

Stiglitz, Joseph E. *The Price of Inequality: How Today's Divided Society Endangers Our Future*. New York: Norton, 2012.

Stoler, Ann Laura. *Carnal Knowledge and Imperial Power: Race and the Intimate in Colonial Rule*. Berkeley: University of California Press, 2002.

Streets, Heather. *Martial Races: The Military, Race and Masculinity in British Imperial Culture, 1857–1914*. Manchester: Manchester University Press, 2011.

Stuart, Tristram. *The Bloodless Revolution: Radical Vegetarians and the Discovery of India*. London: Harper Press, 2006.

Suchitra. "What Moves Masses: Dandi March as Communication Strategy." *Economic and Political Weekly* 30, no. 14 (1995): 743–46.

Suhrud, Tridip. "Emptied of All but Love: Gandhiji's First Public Fast." In *Rethinking Gandhi and Nonviolent Relationality: Global Perspectives*, edited by Debjani Ganguly and John Docker, 66–79. London: Routledge, 2007.

Svoboda, Robert E. *Ayurveda: Life, Health, and Longevity*. New Delhi: Penguin Books India, 1992.

Swan, Maureen. *Gandhi: The South African Experience*. Johannesburg: Ravan Press, 1985.

Swislocki, Mark. *Culinary Nostalgia: Regional Food Culture and the Urban Experience in Shanghai*. Stanford: Stanford University Press, 2009.

Taneja, Anup. *Gandhi, Women, and the National Movement, 1920–47*. New Delhi: Har-Anand, 2005.

Thapar, Suruchi. "Women as Activists; Women as Symbols: A Study of the Indian Nationalist Movement." *Feminist Review* 44 (1993): 81–96.

Tidrick, Kathryn. *Gandhi: A Political and Spiritual Life*. London: I. B. Tauris, 2006.

Tolstoy, Leo. "The First Step." In *Ethical Vegetarianism: From Pythagoras to Peter Singer*, edited by Kerry S. Walters and Lisa Portmes, 97–106. Albany: State University of New York Press, 1999.

———. *The Kingdom of God Is Within You: Christianity Not as a Mystical Doctrine but as a New Understanding of Life*. Radford: Wilder Publications, 2008.

Vajpeyi, Ananya. *Righteous Republic: The Political Foundations of Modern India*. Cambridge, MA: Harvard University Press, 2012.

Valenze, Deborah. *Milk: A Local and Global History*. New Haven: Yale University Press, 2012.

Veit, Helen Zoe. *Modern Food, Moral Food: Self-Control, Science, and the Rise of Modern American Eating in the Early Twentieth Century*. Chapel Hill: University of North Carolina Press, 2013.

Vernon, James. *Hunger: A Modern History*. Cambridge, MA: Harvard University Press, 2007.

Vivekananda, Swami. "Inspired Talks." July 31, 1895. https://sfvedanta.org
/monthly-reading/i-want-to-taste-sugar/.

Vodeb, Oliver, ed. *Food Democracy: Critical Lessons in Food, Communication,
Design and Art.* Chicago: Intellect, 2017.

Warboys, Michael. "The Discovery of Colonial Malnutrition between the Wars."
In *Imperial Medicine and Indigenous Societies,* edited by David Arnold, 208–22.
Manchester: Manchester University Press, 1988.

Weber, Thomas. *Gandhi as Disciple and Mentor.* Cambridge: Cambridge University Press, 2004.

———. *On the Salt March: The Historiography of Gandhi's March to Dandi.* New
Delhi: HarperCollins Publishers India, 1997.

West, Albert. "In the Early Days with Gandhi—I." *Illustrated Weekly of India* 3
(October 1965).Wiley, Andrea S. "Milk for 'Growth': Global and Local
Meanings of Milk Consumption in China, India, and the United States." *Food
and Foodways* 19, nos. 1–2 (2011): 11–33.

Willett, Walter. *Eat, Drink, and Be Healthy: The Harvard Medical School Guide to
Healthy Eating.* New York: Free Press, 2005.

Wilson, A. N. *Tolstoy: A Biography.* New York: Norton, 2001.

Winne, Mark. *Closing the Food Gap: Resetting the Table in the Land of Plenty.*
Boston: Beacon Press, 2009.

———. *Food Rebels, Guerrilla Gardeners, and Smart-Cookin' Mamas: Fighting Back
in an Age of Industrial Agriculture.* Boston: Beacon Press, 2010.

Winson, Anthony. *The Industrial Diet: The Degradation of Food and the Struggle for
Healthy Eating.* New York: New York University Press, 2014.

Wrangham, Richard. *Catching Fire: How Cooking Made Us Human.* New York:
Basic Books, 2009.

Yao, L. H., et al. "Flavonoids in Food and their Health Benefits." *Plant Foods for
Human Nutrition* 59, no. 3 (2004): 113–22.

Zelliot, Eleanor. *Ambedkar's World: The Making of Babasaheb and the Dalit
Movement.* New Delhi: Navayana, 2013.

Zlotnick, Susan. "Domesticating Imperialism: Curry and Cookbooks in Victorian
England." *Frontiers: A Journal of Women Studies* 16, nos. 2–3 (1996): 51–68.

Index

Gandhi, Manilal (son), 8, 21–22, 150, 154

Gandhi, Ramdas (grandson), 27

Ganesha (Ganapati), 39

Ganguly, Debjani, 178

ganthia, 28–29

gardening, 122–23, 129–30, 174

garlic, 112

gender, 18, 80, 165–67

George V, king of England, 3, 15

ghee, 22–23, 66; absent in South African jails, 29, 116–17; replacements for, 83–84, 112–13

ginger, 95–96

Glasse, Hannah, 83

glucose, 145

gluten, 90

goat meat, 46, 61

goat's milk, 47, 65, 67, 72, 102–3; recipe with, 183; vitamins in, 102–3

Gokhale, Gopal Krishna, 109, 129

golpapadi, 27

Graham, Sylvester, 88–89

Great Britain. *See* British Raj; London

green chutney, 117

Gregg, Richard, 102–3

Guha, Ramachandra, 138

Gujarat, 87, 125, 152

Gujarati language, 70–71, 120

gulab jamun, 40

gur (jaggery), 39–40, 85, 112, 117

Guthman, Julie, 12

Hahnemann, Samuel, 105

halva, 28

Harijan (Dalits), 63, 68, 154–58

hartal, 148–49

Hassanein, Neva, 172

Hauter, Wenonah, 136

heating foods, 25, 28, 41, 66

Hills, Arnold, 53, 56, 57

Hind Swaraj (Gandhi), 13, 40, 84, 99, 105, 131

Hinduism, 18, 29, 167, 178; asceticism of, 26, 39, 41; fasting in, 142, 146, 147; gender and, 166; medicine and, 100–101; vegetarianism in, 31, 51, 53

Hindu-Muslim relations, 27, 71, 100–101; diet and, 63–64; partition and, 22, 109, 139, 141–42, 159–61; at Tolstoy Farm, 133

Hobart, Hi'ilei Julia, 30

honey, 40

hot chocolate, 34, 36

housework, 167

hunger and starvation, 30, 42–43, 151–52, 172–75; famine and, 126–28, 136

Ilanga, 129

imperialism. *See* British Raj

indentured labor, 26, 34–35, 66, 164

India: independence of, 22, 139, 141–42; partition of, 22, 109, 139, 141–42, 159–61; Salt Satyagraha in independence movement for, 9–23

Indian cuisine, 28–29, 30–31, 39, 78, 87, 177; regional variety in, 83

Indian National Congress, 9, 15, 70, 106–7, 163

Indian Opinion, 13, 33, 129, 132

indigo, 136–37

interdining, 157–58

intermarriage, 157–58

Irwin, Lord, 14–17

isabgol (psyllium seed husk), 114

Islam, 70; fasting and, 146, 147; medicine and, 100–101; Salt Satyagraha and, 18, 19. *See also* Hindu-Muslim relations

medicine: allopathic (modern), 99, 101, 105–6, 107, 108–9, 111–12; ayurvedic, 23, 100–101, 106–8, 112, 123; expense of, 105, 106, 108; food as, 93, 101, 102, 112, 162; nature cure, 110–16; for poor, 105–6, 108–9, 110–11; soul in, 114, 115; unani, 100–101, 106–7

Mehta, Jeki, 150, 154

Menon, Tangai, 42–43

Merton, Thomas, 72–73

mesul, 27

methi (fenugreek), 113

mhoura, 68

milk, 21, 47–49, 65–73; alternatives to, 67–69, 83–84; chastity and, 65–66; cooperative distribution of, 125–26; digestibility of, 113; Indian consumption of, 61, 70; as metaphor, 70–71; pasteurization of, 86; as public good, 71; self-control and, 65–66; as vital for poor, 70, 72, 116, 125–26. *See also* goat's milk

Miller, Webb, 15

Mintz, Sidney, 26, 82–83, 142

modak, 39

moderation in eating, 7, 40–41, 84, 144, 151

modern (allopathic) medicine, 99, 101, 105–6, 107, 108–9, 111–12

moksha, 7, 44, 168

Moss, Michael, 10

Muslim League, 160

Muslims. *See* Hindu-Muslim relations; Islam

mustard greens (*sarsav*), 98

Naidu, Sarojini, 15, 18

Namboodiripad, E. M. S., 171

Nandy, Ashis, 165–66

nature cure (naturopathy), 110–16; faith and, 114, 115

Nayar, Pramod, 36

neem, 96, 102–3, 110–12, 123

Nehru, Jawaharlal, 11

New England Journal of Medicine, 20

Noakhali, 139–40

noncooperation movement, 153–55

nonviolence. *See ahimsa*

Norton, Marcy, 36

Norwegian Army, 176

nutritionism, 7, 31, 101, 102

Nutrition Research Laboratories, 135

Ohlange Institute, 33, 128–29

Oldfield, Josiah, 53, 56, 64

omega-3 fatty acids, 7, 61, 97, 116, 182

"one meal a day" practice, 151

onions, 58, 66, 112

palasha, 122

paleo diet, 99

papad, 84

Parsis, 175–76

Pasteur, Louis, 86

pasteurization, 86

Patel, Vallabhbhai, 62, 125

patriarchy, 18, 80, 165

peanut butter, 132

peanut milk, 69

peda, 27

peepal trees, 138–39

pellagra, 88

Perfect Way in Diet, The (Kingsford), 48

pharmaceutical drugs, 99

Phoenix Settlement, 129

Polak, Henry, 58

Polak, Millie, 66, 78

Pollan, Michael, 4

poor: diet of, 42–43, 54, 79, 102, 111, 113, 115–16, 118; farmers as, 120, 123, 124–28, 136–37; fasting and, 151–52;

human physiology and, 47, 48; invention of term, 52; of Kellogg, 39; London Vegetarian Society and, 13, 27, 28, 52–53, 56–58, 89; Namboodiripad's criticism of, 171; nonpolemical embrace of, 47–48; nutritional benefits of, 48–50; religious roots of, 31, 50–51, 52, 53–55, 179; restaurants for, 28, 51–53, 54, 58; self-control and, 62; of Tolstoy, 64, 130; at Tolstoy Farm, 133; violent tactics for, 63–64

Vegetarian Society (Manchester), 52

Veit, Helen Zoe, 29

Viola cinerea (*bandafsha*), 108

vital food. *See* raw food

vitamins, 7, 76, 97, 98, 102–4, 117; cooking and, 103–4; diseases from deficiency in, 88; Gandhi's use of term, 102–3

Vivekananda, Swami, 39

voluntary suffering (*tapasya*), 41–42

Wadala Salt Works, 16

Washington, Booker T., 32–33

water: in farming, 173–74; in fasting, 144

Wavell, Lord, 17

West, Albert, 58

Western (allopathic) medicine, 99, 101, 105–6, 107, 108–9, 111–12

What Congress and Gandhi Have Done to the Untouchables (Ambedkar), 157

wheat, 74–75, 86–92, 95, 116; coffee substitute from, 34; rice compared with, 90–91, 104, 136

wheat berry porridge (recipe), 184

Wheel of Life, 135–36

White, E. B., 163

white goosefoot (*chakwat*), 97–98

white South Africans, 32, 128, 150

whole foods, 82, 93

whole grain bread, 84, 88–90, 132

wild food, 97–99, 118; poor and, 97, 98

"wine, women, and meat" avoidance pledge, 51

women: pregnant, diet of, 92; in Salt Satyagraha, 18–19

women's liberation, 18–19, 165–67; raw food in, 80

wood apple (*koth*), 117

Worcestershire sauce, 83, 112

Wrangham, Richard, 76

Yates, May, 89–90

Yeravda jail, 21, 62, 65, 79, 122, 144

yogurt, 73, 113, 181

Zulu Christian Industrial School (Ohlange Institute), 33, 128–29

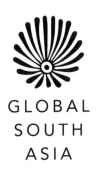

GLOBAL
SOUTH
ASIA

Padma Kaimal, K. Sivaramakrishnan, and Anand A. Yang, Series Editors

Global South Asia takes an interdisciplinary approach to the humanities and social sciences in its exploration of how South Asia, through its global influence, is and has been shaping the world.

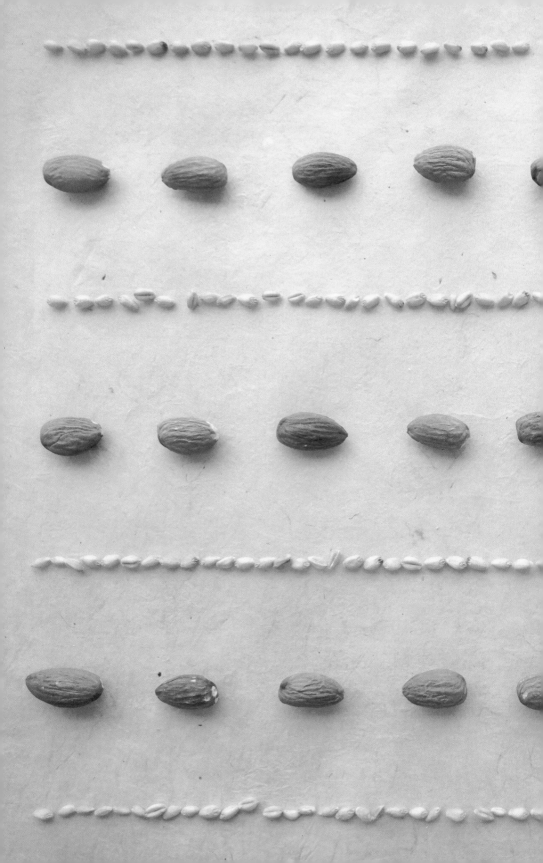